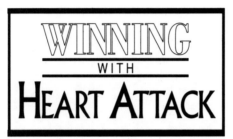

WINNING
WITH
HEART ATTACK

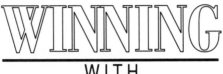

WINNING WITH HEART ATTACK

A Complete Program for Health and Well-Being

*Leading specialists show how you can reduce
or prevent your risk of heart attack.
Vital information on maintaining a healthy heart.*

•

- Learn the latest information about heart attack and its effects
- Rate your risk factors
- Develop your own "heart-healthy" diet
- Get answers to the most frequently asked questions
- Easy to read . . . easy to understand

•

**Harris H. McIlwain, M.D.
Debra Fulghum Bruce
Benedict S. Maniscalco, M.D.
Joel C. Silverfield, M.D.
Michael C. Burnette, M.D.
Bernard F. Germain, M.D.**

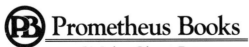 **Prometheus Books**

59 John Glenn Drive
Amherst, New York 14228-2197

Published 1994 by Prometheus Books

98 97 96 95 94   5 4 3 2 1

Library of Congress Cataloging-in-Publication Data

Winning with heart attack : a complete program for health and well-being /
Harris H. McIlwain . . . [et al.].
        p.   cm.
    Includes bibliographical references.
    ISBN 0-87975-914-3 (alk. paper: cloth)
    ISBN 0-87975-915-1 (alk. paper: pbk.)
    1. Myocardial infarction—Popular works. 2. Coronary heart disease—
Popular works. I. McIlwain, Harris H.
RC685.I6W56   1994
616.1'237—dc20   94-25409
                                                               CIP

Printed in the United States of America on acid-free paper.

Acknowledgments

We greatly appreciate the contributions from these professionals who donated time and talents to make *Winning with Heart Attack* complete:

Peter Alagona, Jr., M.D.; Francis I. Barford, L.O.T.R.; Patty Carroscia, R.N.; Dennis M. Cassidy, M.D.; Dana S. Deboskey, Ph.D.; Jewel H. Fulghum; Matthew U. Glover, M.D.; Anthony P. Goldman, M.D.; Susan Haley, R.D., L.D.; Virginia S. Hammond, M.D.; James M. Irwin, M.D.; Suzanne Kesler, A.R.N.P.; Kimberly L. McIlwain; Laura Elizabeth McIlwain; Henry D. McIntosh, M.D.; Dominador U. Martirez, R.P.T., L.P.T.; Medical Library, St. Joseph's Hospital, Tampa, FL; Xavier E. Prida, M.D.; Rick Ruge, Supervisor, Media Services, University Community Hospital, Tampa, Florida; Jeffrey L. Sutton, M.D.; Roger B. Szuch, L.C.S.W.; Tampa Medical Group, P.A.; John C. Toole, M.D.; Vicki K. Windsor, R.P.R.; and Gary Wood, Ph.D.

Contents

1

Start Today to *Win* with Heart Attack

If you are reading this book, chances are great that you or someone you know has suffered a heart attack. Or you may want to take steps to prevent heart attack altogether. Do you know the facts?

- As many as 1.5 million Americans have heart attacks each year and about 500,000 die.

- More than 11 million Americans are affected by coronary heart disease. An even greater number don't know that they have heart problems.

- Sixty million people have high blood pressure, and 80 million have abnormal cholesterol levels, both important risk factors for heart attack.

- Fifty to 100 billion dollars a year are spent to treat heart attack and coronary heart disease, and problems arising from them, including hospitalization, medical tests, and loss of work.

While heart attack is *the number one killer* in the United States, in many cases it can now be prevented! Heart attack does restrict the lives of many, but this condition does not have to be an ordeal. You *can* win the battle with heart attack and live a normal, productive life, taking measures to reduce the chance of further problems.

When we first saw Zack T., now sixty-two, his chances for continuing to live a normal life were quite slim. This successful owner of a car dealership had experienced slight chest pains for several weeks when he exercised or had stress at work. "I thought they would just go away," he told us, "but in the past four days, I have had pain more often with numbness in my left arm."

Zack was admitted to a nearby hospital immediately; after some

1

tests were run, he was found to have coronary heart disease. Zack underwent angioplasty* later that day and was discharged two days later.

When we spoke with Zack in the hospital about his test results, he knew that his destiny was in his own hands: he could ignore the high blood cholesterol, high blood pressure, and continue smoking three packs of cigarettes a day, or he could make some drastic lifestyle changes and begin a program to stop heart attack before it was too late. He vowed to stop cigarettes, began an exercise program for heart patients at the local YMCA, and started eating for a healthy heart instead of "what tasted good." In six months, Zack reduced his chances of heart attack immensely: his blood cholesterol dropped to a safe range under 200 and his blood pressure, now controlled by medication and exercise, was normal. Zack was a new man.

But Zack was also a lucky man! In the past, millions of people have not been as fortunate as Zack in recognizing the early warning signs of heart attack in order to be able to change their lifestyle and control this disease. Using the information given in this book, you can stop heart attack from claiming you as a victim, or at least greatly improve your chances. If you have already had a heart attack, this book will outline a program to change your lifestyle as you reduce the chances of a future attack.

Winning with Heart Attack was written to offer new hope to the millions of people who have already suffered with heart attack or who live in fear of having one. In this book we will tell you how people all around the world are now living active and normal lives—even after having a heart attack. We will offer examples of those who have experienced heart attack and let you know the latest, most effective methods of treatment and prevention.

We will describe people who have many risk factors for heart attack, including a strong family history of heart disease, and show you how they are working to reduce their risk factors, thereby decreasing their chances of heart attack. This book will explain the importance of:

- understanding crucial risk factors for heart attack and learning how to reduce your risk, starting today;

- exercising and following a healthy, low fat diet after heart attack to help prevent future problems;

---

*Angioplasty is performed to reduce the blockage in a coronary artery. See p. 77.

- taking aspirin and vitamin E to help prevent heart attack;

- treating hypertension and high cholesterol, and quitting cigarettes to greatly reduce chances of having heart attack;

- understanding the special risks all women face for heart attack;

- knowing your personality traits and how a type "A" personality increases your risk of heart attack;

- electing surgery as a treatment;

- managing your weight and stress in order to improve your quality of life and reduce your chances of future heart attacks;

- and more!

Winning with Heart Attack will teach you how to prevent more coronary problems as you become active and participate in a full, normal life.

WHAT IS HEART ATTACK?

Heart attack means a blockage of one of the coronary arteries that supply the heart. When this occurs, the blood and oxygen supply to the heart muscle is stopped—the heart muscle may then stop pumping blood to the brain and other vital organs. Or the heart may begin to beat very irregularly. Each of these problems can cause death if not corrected quickly. In fact, the most common cause of death early in a heart attack is from irregular heart beat (see discussion on p. 61).

In many cases, a heart attack is like "the tip of an iceberg." It may be the first overt sign of an underlying heart problem that has been building gradually for years. But given the proper information, you can predict whether you are at higher risk for a heart attack in the future. This information is critical, since it also can allow you to take steps to prevent heart attack altogether.

If you already suffer from coronary heart disease, you may learn the facts from the latest studies that show how the disease can be arrested and its effects even reversed. Thus you can take steps to lower your risk of another heart attack.

HEART ATTACK STARTS
WITH ATHEROSCLEROSIS

The basic problem in most heart attacks is due to *atherosclerosis,* resulting in the narrowing and hardening of the arteries. This process, which builds up over the years, can also cause strokes and heart and kidney failure. These problems are the most common causes of serious illness and death in America. But the leading cause of death is still heart attack.

Researchers think atherosclerosis begins slowly with minor injuries or wear and tear of the inside lining of the arteries, especially the coronary arteries that supply the heart muscle. Normal turbulence of the flow of blood at branches in the arteries, cigarette smoking, and high blood cholesterol may all contribute to these minor injuries (see figure 1.1).

Some think that at the site of a minor injury a reaction by some of the blood cells occurs. This reaction gradually makes the area of injury larger and therefore more likely for a clot to form around that area in the blood vessel. Over time, this builds up and thickens the arterial wall. As time passes, small cracks or fissures form in the same area, which further increase the formation of clots, thus worsening the narrowing of the artery. A larger clot (known as a *thrombosis*) can occur suddenly, partially blocking the flow of blood in the artery or even stopping it altogether. When this happens there are certain signs and symptoms you may experience (see chapter 3).

When blood flow is blocked to the heart muscle, it can become damaged or die, resulting in a heart attack (*myocardial infarction*). When this occurs, heartbeat can become very irregular or the heart muscle may not pump blood to the body's organs, and heart failure may result.

WHO IS AFFECTED BY ATHEROSCLEROSIS?

Of the over 11 million Americans affected by coronary heart disease, more than 1.5 million suffer a heart attack (acute myocardial infarction) each year. One-third of these heart attack victims, or about 500,000 men and women, die each year. Of these who survive heart attack, many are unable to work or have a greatly reduced range of activity.

The amount of health care required increases greatly after a heart attack. This, combined with the loss of work and income places more stress on the patient and family. Medical and other costs resulting from the disease range from $50 to $100 billion a year. Added to this expense is the human cost of suffering among patients and their families. Only

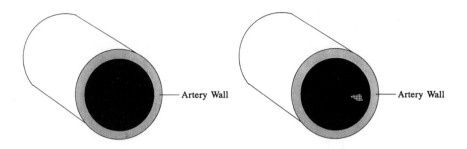

a) Normal artery with no blockage from atherosclerosis.

b) Minor injuries may help start the damage to the wall of the artery.

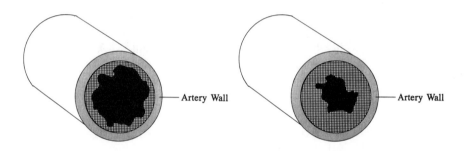

c) The area of injury becomes larger in the artery wall.

d) The thickening gradually increases and narrows the artery.

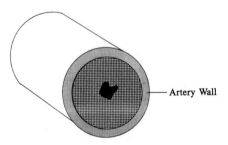

e) Small cracks or fissures can happen which can cause worsening or complete blockage of the artery.

Figure 1.1
Progressive buildup of atherosclerosis in a coronary artery

those families who have experienced heart attack can understand the emotional cost to a loved one disabled by this disease.

HEART ATTACK STOPS YOU IN YOUR TRACKS

Pete H., a 52-year-old father of three teenagers, knows all too well the expense of heart attack. Four years ago, at the height of his career as a self-employed stockbroker, Pete suffered a major heart attack. "Here I was with three kids in college and trying to pay for this without going under," Pete said. "Then . . . bang! I felt the most horrible pain in my chest one day while driving to a brokers' seminar. I knew something serious was happening to my body and drove straight to the emergency room. The rest is heart history for me."

Pete was out of work for several months as he struggled to recuperate. During that time Pete's wife, Nancy, went back to work teaching to help pay for the college tuitions and other living expenses. "A stockbroker who is not dealing with clients cannot make any money," Pete said bluntly. "Those were bad times. I wished I had recognized the risk factors and spent my time doing something to prevent this rather than trying to get well."

When Pete looked over his lifestyle before the heart attack, he realized that he was the right sex and age, smoked cigarettes, had diabetes and high blood pressure, and lived a high-stress life. "I'm in control of my health now," he says, "but it has cost me a great deal of time and money."

Millions of people wish they, too, could turn back the clock and start over. While this is not possible, you can begin today to find out your risks for heart attack, and then do something to eliminate them.

PEOPLE WHO ARE WINNING WITH HEART ATTACK

If you have had a heart attack, don't feel that you have to sit back and allow your life to pass you by. Let's look at some case studies of people who have taken control of their health and are living quite normal lives after heart attack.

Bill R. was a 55-year-old auto parts manager when he first found out about heart disease. "I had developed pain and stiffness in my left hip due to arthritis," Bill told us, "so to improve the strength of my stiff hip, I began using an exercise bicycle. After a few weeks, I noticed some tightness in my chest when I pedaled the bike. The tightness went away when I rested. After a few times experiencing this new feeling, I checked with my doctor to be sure nothing was wrong."

Bill told of having tests showing major blockage of two of his coronary arteries. He then had angioplasty, correcting the blockage without surgery.

"Since my angioplasty, I have resumed riding my exercise bicycle," Bill continued. "I even play golf twice a week, and have had no problems or limitations over the past nine years." Bill still works full-time and even took over ownership of the auto parts store. It is very likely that Bill prevented a serious and possibly fatal heart attack by taking the right steps early.

Michael P., a 62-year-old insurance salesman, had known for years that he suffered from heart disease. "I depended on nitroglycerin tablets when I had chest pain and remained active as a grandfather, taking the kids on trips each weekend," Michael said. "One day I collapsed while shopping at the mall with my oldest grandson; my heart completely stopped. Luckily, my grandson was there to call for help. A nurse who was shopping nearby, ran over and quickly began CPR [cardiopulmonary resuscitation]."

Michael was taken to a nearby hospital, where it was found that his heart had a very unstable rhythm, putting him continuously at risk for cardiac arrest (i.e., the sudden stopping of his heart). A special device was inserted which automatically corrected the irregularity whenever it occurred. Two years have passed now with no further problems, and Michael continues to enjoy his life as a grandfather.

Mary Louise B. was sixty years old when she first experienced chest pain. Mary Louise had known about hypertension, or high blood pressure, for years, and she was familiar with heart disease because her father had died of a heart attack. "I had severe pain early one morning which woke me up suddenly," she told us. "It felt like a fire was burning in the center of my chest. I then became extremely short of breath and sweaty; I knew something was wrong."

Mary Louise was taken by her husband to an emergency room where she was diagnosed as having had a heart attack. After later tests showed severe blockage of three coronary arteries, coronary bypass surgery was performed. This was seven years ago, and since that time Mary Louise has done well, walking several miles daily as part of her exercise program and even playing doubles tennis with her friends.

Randall C. had his first heart attack at the young age of forty-nine. "I had some chest pain after playing softball at the church picnic one Sunday afternoon," he said. "I thought I had pulled a muscle, but it would not go away. By the time I got home that night, it felt as if an elephant had planted itself on my chest and would not move. I was sweating profusely, and began to vomit. Everything was spinning around in front of me, and I was in so much pain. Then I knew it wasn't a pulled muscle, and my wife called 911 for an ambulance."

After Randall got to the hospital, he was diagnosed with heart attack. He stayed in the intensive care for three days, then was moved to a private room. When Randall finally got home, he began to evaluate his risk factors for heart attack with the attending physician. "I certainly had almost every risk factor on the list," he told us. "My father and older brother both had heart attacks at an early age, I smoked two packs of cigarettes a day, my cholesterol was well over 200, and I rarely exercised."

Randall decided then to take control of his health and eliminate all the risk factors he could for heart attack. He quit smoking that very day, began a high complex carbohydrate, low fat diet, and started to walk each day, building up to two miles daily within two months. Although Randall's family history still puts him at risk for heart attack, he has now taken charge of his life and is doing all he can to reduce the other risk factors.

Sharon T. is another lucky person who survived a heart attack when she was only fifty-one years old! "My family history must be against me," she said. "Both my parents had heart attacks before the age of fifty, and so did my older brother. I always thought that because I was a female, it would never happen to me. And I tried to do everything right—exercise every day and never smoke—but it was not enough."

Sharon was playing tennis on the women's team at a local club when she noticed her left arm feeling very heavy. "At first I thought I had sprained it from swinging too hard because I am left-handed," she told us. "Then when the heaviness turned to numbness and severe pain spread up into my shoulder, I knew I was having trouble."

Sharon went immediately to a nearby emergency room; after some tests, she was prepped for angioplasty later that afternoon. "I had a major blockage in the coronary arteries, just like my parents and brother had," she said. Unlike her parents and brother, who had died of heart attack, Sharon was lucky that the angioplasty corrected the problem; she was back on the courts within weeks. But she also made some careful lifestyle changes to reduce her high risk of heart attack.

"Even though I exercised daily, I still had a very poor diet," Sharon said. "I simply ate too much fat. I have learned to eat the right way, reducing my fat to about 15 percent of my total calories. With this diet and some cholesterol-lowering medication, my cholesterol (which was over 250) has come down to around 180, within the safe range. Because of my family history, I am now staying close to my doctor to keep check on my heart, but now I feel like I am in control."

YOU *CAN* WIN WITH HEART ATTACK

Yes, you, too, can win with heart attack and other heart disease caused by narrowing and hardening of the arteries that supply the heart. Even though heart attack is the most common cause of death in America, there are easy ways to lower your chances and even prevent an attack altogether. There are also ways to control the disease after a heart attack in order to allow you to become active and pain-free.

The most effective plan is to take steps to prevent the start or the progression of arterial disease. Research has shown that prevention of heart attacks and second heart attacks is possible. You can do this by taking specific steps, such as controlling cholesterol, cutting out cigarettes, and changing your activity to include exercise. These actions are not difficult once you know about them. And many studies show that these simple treatments can make a difference in whether a second heart attack will happen. Just think! Simply by making some changes in the foods you eat and the way you spend your free time, you could ultimately change your life as you become aware of heart-healthy eating, exercising for a strong heart, saying no to cigarettes, and more.

In one-third of all cases, heart attack is the first overt sign of a heart problem, even though in most cases strong risk factors are present which could have warned of the danger. Sadly, many of the half million American men and women at risk who die each year of a heart attack might have been saved if precautions had been taken earlier.

RISK FACTORS INCREASE THE CHANCES OF HEART ATTACK

Certain risk factors can greatly raise one's chances for heart attack. For example, between 50 and 60 million Americans have blood pressure high enough to raise their risk of heart attack. This condition, known as hypertension, increases the risk of heart attack in men, but it's especially serious for women. It has been estimated that at least 10 percent of deaths from coronary heart disease each year could be prevented simply by treating hypertension. This means that perhaps 50,000 needless deaths might be avoided annually! In other words, see your doctor if you are at risk; and if you are diagnosed with hypertension, take your medication, as directed, each day. Control your blood pressure—and along with it greatly reduce your chance of heart attack. Reducing blood pressure to normal levels also lowers the chance of stroke by reducing damage to blood vessels in the brain.

Randy P., a 49-year-old school teacher, didn't know he had high blood pressure until a paramedic was showing his students how to use the pressure monitor. "The young man checked the blood pressure of several students, then he took mine," Randy said. "When he called out the numbers of 160/102, I knew I had a problem."

Randy came to our clinic after school that day and got his blood pressure checked again. It was lower at that reading, but still in a high range. After several subsequent readings that were equally as high, Randy started on medication to reduce his blood pressure. He has been on this medication for five years now and is able to keep his pressure normal with a healthy diet and active exercise program. Randy's other risk factors for heart attack are low in that he does not smoke, has a cholesterol level of 172, walks daily, controls his stress in a beneficial manner, and has no history of heart attack in his family.

ABNORMAL CHOLESTEROL

About 80 million Americans suffer from high blood cholesterol, which also increases the risk of heart attack. For example, the risk of heart attack has been found to increase when cholesterol levels are above 200 mg/dl (milligrams per deciliter). The risk doubles in both men and women if the cholesterol level is above 240–265 (see pp. 24–25).

Actually, most heart attacks occur with the total cholesterol level between 200 and 240 ("borderline high"), although about 15 percent of heart attacks happen to people whose total cholesterol falls below 200 ("normal"). You don't have to let elevated cholesterol be a risk factor in your life. You can begin today to control your cholesterol (see chapter 5), thus lowering your risk of heart attack.

One patient, Lucy S., the busy owner of a women's retail shop, told of having to relearn how to eat. "No one likes to eat more than I do," she told us. "In the past, I loved parties and mixed drinks. After work each day, I used to come home and snack on cheese and crackers before having a heavy dinner around 9:00 P.M. I just didn't have time to go to the market and buy fresh vegetables. Instead, I relied on the deli down the street from my shop for breakfast and lunch. But what I was putting in my mouth was totally poisoning my body."

After finding out that her cholesterol levels were well over 200, Lucy knew she had to find time to change her diet. "It hasn't been easy, but I keep a refrigerator and small microwave in the back room of the shop. I buy a lot of healthy low-fat, low-sodium prepared frozen dinners for lunch, and I eat no-fat cereals or bagels and fruit for breakfast. It took some getting used to, but after six months, my cholesterol has dropped 40 points and is getting closer to 200. I've even lost fourteen pounds since I started this. I think I am in control now."

Take advantage of the opportunities you have to control your risk factors for heart attack by knowing your cholesterol level and blood pressure.

HEART ATTACK IS *NOT* FOR MEN ONLY

Heart attack strikes both men and women. Between the ages of thirty-five and forty-four, coronary heart disease is much more common in men than women—at least six times more common. But after menopause, heart attacks among women begin to increase as estrogen levels decrease (see p. 45). In fact, by age sixty-five, women equal men in the rate of heart attacks.

As we get older, the risk of death from heart attack increases for all of us. Eighty percent of deaths due to heart attack occur in persons sixty-five or older, and most of these actually occur after age seventy-five. Since there are more women than men alive after age seventy-five, heart attacks during these years occur predominantly among women. In fact, at least 250,000 women of all ages die each year of heart attacks, making it the leading cause of death for women today! Coronary heart disease is also the most common cause of disability in women, as well as one of the most common reasons for admission to a hospital for older women.

Women should be aware that once heart disease strikes, there are times they may actually be at higher risk than men regardless of age.

For example, studies have found that the chance of death early after a heart attack is higher in women than men. Also, the chance of death in a hospital is higher among women than men after coronary bypass surgery.

The reasons behind these occurrences are not known. Some researchers have suggested that more severe disease or delay in care might account for some of the difference. But it is known that in previous years, the use of certain tests to discover heart disease were less commonly done with women than with men. These include some of the tests to be discussed in chapter 4, such as coronary arteriogram (where dye is injected into the coronary arteries to find any blockage). To find and treat heart disease at the earliest possible time, when treatment may be most effective, women must know the facts and be comfortable in the knowledge that their own problems are being given attention. Talk with your doctor about your individual problems and needs, and make sure that something is being done to diagnose and treat any heart condition.

The program described in this book will help men, women and their families lower the risk of future heart attack by controlling risk factors years earlier in life—even in childhood (see chapter 5). Even as you get older, you can still lower your chance for heart attack by detection and elimination or control of risk factors.

TAKE CHARGE OF YOUR HEART

Yes, you can manage the problem of coronary heart disease if you know what to do. The steps can be clear once you have talked with your doctor and made a plan, using the steps described in this book. Millions of persons who suffer a heart attack have been able to make needed changes and go on to live active, healthy, and long lives.

Can you take charge of your own prevention and treatment program in coronary heart disease? It is possible to change the problem from terrible and life-threatening to manageable. Most of all, don't become discouraged and don't panic. Men and women should learn the facts and make a plan.

After seeing his doctor for an ankle injury six years ago, Scott A. had to make some hard choices. "My doctor looked at me and told me that I would probably not live to see my fiftieth birthday," Scott said. "I couldn't believe it! I was only forty-six years old and in perfect health, or so I thought. I bowled twice a week on my work team and hardly ever drank."

But Scott's doctor saw the familiar warning signs: "He did some routine tests and called me immediately," Scott said. "My cholesterol was over 300, my blood pressure was high, and I absolutely had to quit smoking cigarettes. I was overweight, and even though I thought I was in control, stress was getting the best of me."

"The doctor left it up to me," Scott continued. "I had to make some life choices that were not easy."

To stop smoking Scott went to a clinic sponsored by the American Lung Association, and with the help of his physician and a prescription nicotine patch, he was able to quit cigarettes for good. He began a walking and exercise program, starting with just two blocks and working up to three miles a day, four days a week. After several weeks, Scott and his wife, Marie, took a nutrition course offered at a local wellness center and began to experiment with low-fat cooking, keeping their total calorie intake per day to under 20 percent fat.

"It actually became fun to see how healthy we could eat," Scott said. "Instead of fried foods, we baked skinless chicken or grilled our fish. We ate salads, fresh vegetables and fruits, and whole grain breads. Marie began to walk with me in the evening, and this was a special time for us. But the greatest reward was at my physical two years later. My blood pressure was normal, my cholesterol had dropped to 180, and I had not smoked cigarettes for twenty-three months. I took charge of my health and my heart, and I'm alive and well today because of this."

Scott, now a much healthier 52-year-old, forgot to mention that his bowling score improved as well! Like Scott, all women and men should look at their own risk factors and know that most of these can be changed to prevent heart attack or prevent worsening of coronary heart disease.

FROM PATIENT TO PERSON

For those who have suffered with heart attack, there is hope. Heart attack can be treated, and you can begin to live a normal life. The best hope is to eliminate the risk factors and prevent heart attack altogether, but in many cases this simply cannot be done.

However, it is now known that most of those who suffer from heart attack can benefit greatly from lifestyle changes, including exercise programs, quitting cigarettes, weight reduction, low-fat and high complex carbohydrate diets, stress management, controlling hypertension and cholesterol, and more. It is not necessary to live with the fear of more problems; it is possible to live a normal life, engaging in the activities you choose.

The main ingredient in the treatment and prevention of heart attack is you—*if* you begin a comprehensive program to eliminate risk factors. In other words, you can change things in your life so that the chances of having a heart attack are greatly reduced. You can begin to live your life again and move from being "patient" to "person"—to happier times at home and improved quality times at work and play—without the nagging fear of heart attack.

Let's get started.

2

Rating Your Risk Factors

Risk factors play a vital part in the prevention of many diseases. Just as there are various risk factors that affect one's chances of developing cancer, osteoporosis, or diabetes, so are there also important factors to consider for heart attack. Even though their exact causes are not known, specific risk factors definitely increase the likelihood of a heart attack (see table 2.1). When these problems are identified, you can begin to take control in order to remove or greatly reduce these risk factors, thereby lowering your chances of heart attack.

In dealing with heart attack, the very best treatment is prevention altogether of atherosclerosis and narrowing of the coronary arteries. But even if heart disease is already present, much can still be done to stop or ameliorate the blockage in the arteries and to help prevent future heart attack and, possibly, death.

For example, a 50-year-old American man who smokes cigarettes and has high blood pressure (hypertension) runs a risk of heart attack about five times the national average. Simply by stopping cigarettes or controlling blood pressure, this man can lower his risk of heart attack. Men who smoke and have hypertension and high blood cholesterol run a risk about twenty times the national average for heart attack!

PEOPLE AFFECTED BY HEART ATTACK

Ron A. is a 69-year-old man with a strong family history of heart disease. All three of his brothers died from heart attack, two before age fifty and one at age sixty. Ron was fifty-three when his third brother died, and at that time, Ron smoked over two packs of cigarettes a day, worked a high-stress job, and was overweight.

Realizing the seriousness of his family history of heart disease, Ron began a program to quit smoking, lose weight, and control stress. He started walking each day before going to work, changed his diet to include many fruits and vegetables, and limited saturated fats. Sixteen years later, Ron enjoys his retirement with his wife and grandchildren. Given his strong family history for heart attack, if Ron had continued smoking, eating the wrong foods, and maintaining his high-stress lifestyle, his chances for developing heart problems would have been much greater.

Mick T. was forty-nine years old when he began treatment for high blood pressure. "High blood pressure runs in my family," Mick told us, "and I have seen what can happen if you let it go untreated. Not only do I take my medicine, but I walk three miles at least four times a week to keep my pressure low. I want to do all I can to reduce this risk factor."

Walking combined with medication can be an important part of the treatment for high blood pressure. Some people are able to reduce their medication when they stay on an exercise program, and some have even been able to stop medication completely as their blood pressure has remained low due to regular exercise and a heart-healthy diet.

Table 2.1
Risk Factors for Heart Attack

1. High blood pressure (hypertension)

2. High blood cholesterol (hypercholesterolemia)

3. Cigarette smoking

4. Poor diet

5. Lack of exercise

6. Being overweight

7. Stress

8. Personality traits—hostility and anger

9. Sex and menopause

10. Increasing age

11. Diabetes mellitus

12. Family history of heart disease

PLOT YOUR COURSE WITH HEART ATTACK

It is not necessary to just "hope" that you don't eventually have a heart attack. You can put your destiny in good hands as you predict your own chances of having heart attack. Looking at the risk factors listed in table 2.1 can help determine your own risk. If you have no classic risk factors, then your chances for heart attack and other problems from atherosclerosis are low. However, you should continue to keep your cholesterol levels and blood pressure low; stay away from cigarettes; eat a healthy, low-fat diet; and exercise. Even if you do have some risk factors, then you can begin to change or eliminate them and thus lower your heart attack risk!

On the following pages you will find described the most common risk factors already outlined for heart attack and atherosclerosis. Take a few minutes to review these and see how they relate to your life. Simply checking these once a year can give great returns on a small investment of time. For example, if your blood pressure happens to be high, it is an easy problem to solve, thereby reducing your risk of heart attack by half!

In fact, over the past twenty years there has been a 45 to 50 percent decrease in heart attacks and a 57 percent decrease in strokes in the U.S. This reduction can be largely attributed to better control of hypertension.

Let's now discuss the most common factors that can increase the likelihood of heart attack and other problems caused by atherosclerosis. Check to see which ones are present in your own case—and then discover how easy it can be to remove those risks.

RISK FACTORS THAT LEAD TO HEART ATTACK

1. Hypertension

High blood pressure increases the risk for heart attack and other problems caused by atherosclerosis. The higher the blood pressure, the higher the risk. Insurance companies know that if clients' blood pressure is high, they have a greater chance of dying prematurely. Generally, hypertension increases the risk of heart attack and coronary heart disease by about *50 percent* in men and may increase the risks *fourfold* in women.

Some research has found that damage from blood pressure gradually increases above readings of 120/80. Seventy to 80 percent of men and women in the United States have blood pressure higher than this figure! (Normal blood pressure is less than 130/85.)

Therefore, if your blood pressure is up, you are *not* alone: 50 to 60 million Americans have blood pressure readings higher than 140/90. Two-thirds of these have diastolic (the lower number) blood pressure between 90 and 104. Hypertension is three times more common in African Americans than in whites. Also, if you have a family member with hypertension, your own risk is thereby higher.

Blood Pressure Can Increase With Age

Fifty percent or more of men and women over age sixty-five may be found to have hypertension. Between the ages of sixty-five and seventy-four it is more common in African Americans than whites and more often found in women than men.

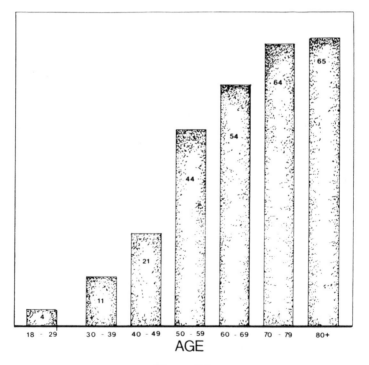

Figure 2.1
Percentage of Americans with hypertension, according to age

Source: Centers for Disease Control, National Center for Health Statistics, *Third National Health and Nutrition Examination Survey, 1988-91.*

Measure Your Blood Pressure

You don't have to wonder what your blood pressure is; it's easy to find out. There are many convenient locations where you can check it regularly—at your doctor's office, fire stations, grocery stores, pharmacies, and shopping malls.

Blood pressure is measured in millimeters of mercury (mm Hg). Two measurements make up the blood pressure. The upper number is the *systolic* blood pressure and the lower number is the *diastolic* blood pressure. Usually the "mm Hg" is eliminated and the blood pressure is said to be "120 over 80" or written 120/80.

The size of the blood pressure cuff itself (that portion you wrap around your arm) should be correct. If your arm is too large for the cuff, it may make the blood pressure appear to be elevated even if it is normal. You then need to use the larger size cuff. Markings on the cuff itself will show if your arm size needs the larger cuff. Cuff-type blood pressure measurements are most common and are usually reliable. If your reading is too high or too low, check with your doctor.

Before checking your blood pressure, sit for a few minutes. Don't check your pressure if you have been smoking, drinking coffee or other caffeine products, taking a common cold medication, or been under stress, which can all raise the blood pressure temporarily. Remember that blood pressure can vary. The body has a normal variation in blood pressure. Readings are usually higher in the early morning and lower in the afternoon.

Reading your blood pressure about every two weeks or so will give you a good idea of your usual pressure. Blood pressure can be measured accurately at home with inexpensive devices available at pharmacies or medical supply stores. Taking your blood pressure at home can allow you to make more readings at different times. Many people find their blood pressure is lower when they measure it at home. It would be a good idea to write your pressure down so that you can see if it changes in the future. Try to check your blood pressure in a sitting position at least twice a year if it remains normal, or more often if it is 130 or higher systolic (upper) or 85 or higher diastolic (lower).

White Coat Hypertension

Some persons may find that they have "white coat" hypertension. In other words, the patient's blood pressure is elevated in the doctor's office or clinic but normal at home or at other times. Measuring the blood pressure outisde the doctor's office can help discover this discrepancy and thus eliminate unnecessary treatment. It is also possible to wear a simple blood pressure monitor that automatically measures pressure during the day and night to obtain a more accurate reading.

The Feelings of High Blood Pressure

How do you feel if your blood pressure is high? Almost always there are *no* unusual feelings. At very high levels there may be headaches or dizziness but it is not safe to expect feelings to help you decide your blood pressure. It must be measured to be accurate.

Normal Blood Pressure

"Normal" blood pressure was for years considered to be 140/85 or lower because it was thought that these readings were safe. Researchers have now shown that cardiovascular disease may gradually increase as blood pressure rises above 120/80.

As blood pressure rises above this level, so does the risk of heart disease. This means that over 70 percent of men and up to 80 percent of women over age thirty-five in the United States who have blood pressure over 120/80 may be at higher risk! Control of mild and moderate hypertension (stages 1 and 2: see below) has been shown to lower the risk of coronary heart disease after less than six years of treatment. Long-term control of hypertension may lower overall coronary heart disease by 20 to 25 percent.

When to Get Treatment

If your systolic blood pressure is 130–139 or higher or your diastolic blood pressure is 85–89, you should recheck the measurement at least evey few months to be sure these high normal blood pressures do not become higher.

If, after several readings, your diastolic blood pressure is 85 or higher, or if your systolic blood pressure is 140 or higher, you should check with your doctor and read chapter 5 for treatment possibilities with and without medication.

It used to be thought that systolic blood pressure was not important. Now we know that systolic blood pressure may even be more crucial than diastolic as a contributor to heart disease.

Borderline Systolic Hypertension

Recent evidence has shown that even if your systolic blood pressure is between 140 and 160, and your diastolic pressure is less than 90, treatment may still be needed. This "borderline" systolic hypertension may gradually increase to definite hypertension, which will in turn increase the risk of heart disease. Some studies have found that about 80 percent of these "borderline" cases in men and women turn into "real" hypertension after ten to twenty years. But this borderline condition may itself bring risk for heart disease and death. It is now included in stage 1 (mild) hypertension as discussed below. Follow-up, as in stage 1 hypertension and treatment as outlined in chapter 5 are needed.

Stage 1 (Mild Hypertension)

If your systolic blood pressure is 140–159 *or* your diastolic blood pressure is 90–99, you have stage 1 (mild) hypertension. If several different measurements confirm this reading, then check with your doctor and read pp. 83ff. for steps for treatment without medication. Check your blood pressure at least once every one to two months, and be sure to follow up as outlined on p. 92.

Stage 2 (Moderate Hypertension)

If your systolic blood pressure is 160–179 *or* your diastolic blood pressure is 100–109, you have stage 2 (moderate) hypertension. If repeated measurements confirm this to be accurate, check with your doctor and begin steps for treatment without medication. Check your blood pressure at regular intervals at least several times per month until it becomes more controlled. It would be helpful to be able to measure blood pressure at home or work. If the pressure does not improve within a few months, treatment with medication is warranted.

Stage 3 (Severe Hypertension)

If your systolic blood pressure is 180–209 *or* your diastolic blood pressure is 110–119 then you have stage 3 (severe) hypertension. Check with your doctor as soon as possible, begin the steps for treatment without medication, and follow your doctor's advice about taking medication. Recheck your blood pressure at least every few days until it becomes controlled. It would be helpful to be able to measure your blood pressure at home or work.

Stage 4 (Very Severe Hypertension)

If your systolic blood pressure is 210 or higher *or* your diastolic blood pressure is 120 or higher, then you have stage 4 (very severe) hypertension. *It is extremely important to get medical care immediately.* Call your doctor or go to the nearest emergency medical facility. Begin medication as your doctor advises, start the steps for treatment without medication, and recheck your blood pressure as often as your doctor suggests. This is a very serious medical problem.

Table 2.2
Categories of Hypertension*

	Systolic (upper number)		*Diastolic* (lower number)
Normal Blood Pressure	less than 130		less than 85
High normal	130–139	or	85–89
Hypertension			
Stage 1 (mild)	140–159	or	90–99
Stage 2 (moderate)	160–179	or	100–109
Stage 3 (severe)	180–209	or	110–119
Stage 4 (very severe)	210 or higher	or	120 or higher

Since every person is different, the exact level of high blood pressure needing treatment should be decided with your doctor. Your doctor can also help you decide if any other tests might be needed. Treatment can be successful *without* medications; if necessary, medications should be added. Good control of hypertension can make a major difference in reducing many future medical complications. Indeed, it may be your most important investment in time and effort.

2. High Blood Cholesterol (Hypercholesterolemia)

Cholesterol is normally present in the blood. When the body produces too much, or when levels are too high from other causes, the risk of coronary

*This table shows the categories of hypertension of the Joint National Committee on Detection, Evaluation, and Treatment of High Blood Pressure.

heart disease increases accordingly. This is because high cholesterol levels contribute to the development of atherosclerosis in the walls of the arteries generally but especially in the coronary arteries (see figure 2.2).

The entire process takes years, but may begin with minor irritations and injuries to the wall of an artery, even injury from the turbulent flow of blood. Minor injuries cause tiny breaks on the inside of the lining of the wall of an artery. Then there is a reaction in that area from blood cells and other blood proteins. The reaction causes the wall of the artery to thicken and the artery to become narrower. The thickened walls of the arteries actually contain cholesterol deposits; the higher the cholesterol level in the blood, the greater the chance this process will occur.

A blood clot may form around the tiny cracks in these abnormal areas and may completely block the flow of blood. These clots, which may occur suddenly, are a common cause of heart attacks.

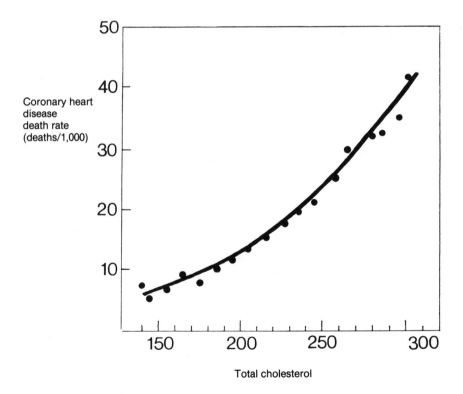

Figure 2.2
The risk of heart attack increases along with the total cholesterol.

"Normal" Cholesterol

"Normal" total cholesterol level is considered to be that below 200 mg/dl (see table 2.3). However, up to half of patients who have already had a heart attack, coronary artery bypass, or angioplasty may have cholesterol levels in this "normal" range if other types of cholesterol are not measured. The risk of heart attack increases gradually as the total cholesterol level increases above 200. Fifty to 80 percent of men in some studies have cholesterol levels higher than this. Testing for high-density lipoprotein (HDL) cholesterol and low-density lipoprotein (LDL) cholesterol (see below) is also needed.

Table 2.3
Total Cholesterol

If your number is:	*Your level is:*
less than 200*	desirable
200–239	borderline high
240 or higher	high

"Borderline High" Cholesterol

A total blood cholesterol level of 200–240 is called "borderline high." About 30 percent of adults in the United States have cholesterol levels in this range. Even though this range is called borderline, it is the level of cholesterol found in most persons who develop coronary heart disease and heart attack! Further testing for HDL cholesterol and LDL cholesterol (discussed below) is needed when the total cholesterol is 200–240. In some cases, the cholesterol level may be over 200 and still be normal *if* the "good" HDL cholesterol is increased—read on!

"High" Cholesterol

A total cholesterol count above 240 is considered "high." About 20 percent of adults have a cholesterol level above 240. A man whose total cholesterol level is more than 240 runs twice the risk of heart attack as compared to one whose cholesterol is 200. And studies show

---

*This level may vary and still be desirable, depending on HDL cholesterol and LDL cholesterol.

that in women, a total cholesterol level over 265 mg/dl raises the risk of coronary heart disease two to three times as compared to women whose cholesterol is 200 or less. But further testing is needed, since even though the total cholesterol is high, the results can be misleading. What matters is how much of the cholesterol is "good" or "bad."

LDL "Bad" Cholesterol

Cholesterol and other fats in the blood do not circulate alone, but are attached to a protein. The most common protein attached to cholesterol is low-density lipoprotein (LDL). Most of the total blood cholesterol is found in LDL cholesterol. The higher the LDL cholesterol, the greater the risk of heart attack. Because of this, LDL cholesterol has been called the "bad" cholesterol.

The goal for LDL cholesterol should be less than 130 in persons with *no known coronary heart disease*. This is to *prevent* the development of heart disease. LDL cholesterol between 130 and 159 is "borderline high" but does elevate your risk as the level increases. LDL cholesterol of 160 mg/dl or greater doubles the risk of coronary heart disease (see table 2.4). Treatment with diet is discussed on pp. 98ff.

The goal for LDL cholesterol in those who *already have coronary heart disease* is stricter: it should be less than 100 in order to try to *stop* or *reverse* the process. Treatment with diet and medication to achieve these goals is discussed on p. 102.

Table 2.4
LDL Cholesterol: Know Your Number

If your number is:	*The range is:*	*Your risk for heart attack:*
less than 130 mg/dl	normal and desirable	normal
130–160	borderline high	increased
over 160	high	double
less than 100	desirable (if you already have coronary heart disease)	decreased

HDL "Good" Cholesterol

Another protein in the blood that carries cholesterol is high-density lipoprotein (HDL), which contains about 20 percent of the total cholesterol. HDL cholesterol has been found to protect against, and actually *lower,* the risk of heart attack, so it has been called the "good cholesterol."

Researchers have found that cholesterol deposits are removed or prevented from going into the wall of the arteries by HDL cholesterol. This may help explain in part how it can help stop or improve the blockage in coronary arteries.

Women have less coronary heart disease than men from the age of twenty to between fifty and sixty. During this time before menopause, women have higher HDL cholesterol levels than men and have protection against heart disease. Following menopause, when the HDL level becomes lower in women, there is less protective effect and the rate of coronary heart disease thereby increases. By age sixty-five, the rate of heart disease in women catches up with that in men.

When HDL cholesterol drops below 35, there is a higher risk of heart attack. This may explain in part why some persons with apparently normal total cholesterol levels of less than 200 develop heart disease. Studies show that over 10 percent of Americans may have HDL cholesterol below 35.

A desirable level of HDL cholesterol to help lower the risk of heart disease is 60 or higher. This is especially important in those who already have coronary heart disease. As discussed on pp. 104–105, physical activity and moderate amounts of alcohol are good ways to help raise the HDL cholesterol. Cutting out cigarettes, changing the type of fat you eat, and reducing body weight are also ways to help raise the HDL cholesterol.

The key: *lowering* the LDL cholesterol level and *raising* the HDL cholesterol level help prevent heart attack. It is helpful to control cholesterol levels—even in those persons who have already had a heart attack and developed severe coronary heart disease.

Table 2.5
HDL Cholesterol

If your number is:	*Your risk for heart attack is:*
less than 35	higher
over 60	lower

Treatment for High Cholesterol

Don't be discouraged if you have already had a heart attack. Studies show that it is not too late to treat and improve your condition. Research now indicates that the blockage of the arteries can be slowed or even reversed when cholesterol is reduced to effective levels. If you have had coronary bypass surgery or angioplasty (discussed on p. 77), you should plan to prevent the *next* heart attack. There is now proof that reducing cholesterol can work!

Studies have shown that with treatment, including combinations of diet, exercise, and medications, the coronary disease blockage can be slowed or actually reversed. For example, research has revealed that two or three times fewer new blockages developed when high cholesterol was controlled. It is clear—lowering cholesterol in heart disease patients can result in fewer heart attacks and deaths.

Triglycerides Are Important

Others types of fats in the blood are *triglycerides.* These have been thought for years to be less important in causing heart attack unless they become extremely high. Researchers now think that the desirable goal for triglycerides is lower than 200 mg/dl. In certain patients treatment may be needed to bring the level to at least below 250.

There is evidence that high triglycerides increase the risk for coronary heart disease in women. Certain studies have found that middle-aged men and women are both at higher risk for heart disease if triglycerides are high. The combination of high triglycerides and low HDL cholesterol seems responsible for raising such risk.

Table 2.6
Triglycerides

If your number is:	*Your triglycerides are:*
less than 200 mg/dl	desirable
201–249	borderline high
250 or higher	high, treatment considered

Measure Your Cholesterol

A blood test is taken to measure the *total* cholesterol (which should usually be below 200 mg/dl). This test can be taken at any time, whether or not you have eaten. If your total cholesterol is 200 or greater, then repeat a blood test after *fasting* (no food for twelve hours) within eight weeks. The repeat test should include total cholesterol, LDL cholesterol, HDL cholesterol, and triglycerides since all of these can be important in raising or lowering the risk of heart attack. It is also a good idea to check your HDL cholesterol, LDL cholesterol, and triglyceride levels yearly even if your total cholesterol is 200 or less. If your levels are too high, at least two or three different testings should be done in order to determine the true levels so that appropriate treatment may be given.

It has been recommended that all adults over age twenty be tested for blood cholesterol every five years. However, the cost would be hundreds of millions of dollars if all young, middle-aged, and older adults followed this recommendation. Treatment would increase the cost to perhaps billions of dollars. Future research will tell, hopefully, who should be tested more regularly and who may need it less often. Even so, treatment of abnormal cholesterol levels and prevention of heart disease is much cheaper in the long run than treatment of heart attack!

An alternative might be to teach the general population more than they already know about better eating habits to produce lower cholesterol levels. It is easy and should start at an early age, even childhood. If you find your cholesterol to be high, take steps with diet as discussed on pp. 98ff., and, if necessary, use medication to bring your cholesterol to normal levels. Reducing your risk and preventing heart attack will save unnecessary suffering and reduce health care costs.

Treatment Does Work!

Simply follow the steps recommended by the National Cholesterol Education Program. Remember: The main goals of treatment are to *lower* the LDL cholesterol level to normal and to *raise* the HDL cholesterol level.

3. Cigarette Smoking

Smoking raises the risk of coronary heart disease and heart attack. It is especially dangerous in those who also suffer from hypertension or high blood cholesterol. For example, with all three of these factors, the risk of heart disease is twenty times higher than for a nonsmoker who has normal blood pressure and cholesterol levels. The risk of heart disease is five times higher for a person who smokes and has high blood cholesterol. The good news is that by quitting cigarettes, you can quickly lower your chance of heart attack.

Over the years, substances in cigarette smoke increase the risk of heart attack by increasing atherosclerosis, with gradual narrowing and blockage of the coronary arteries. This may happen because smoking lowers HDL (the "good") cholesterol, which helps prevent heart attack by removing or preventing cholesterol deposits in the walls of arteries. Also, because of their direct effect on the artery, cigarettes increase the chance of a sudden clot with major blockage of a coronary artery and subsequent heart attack.

Even a Few Cigarettes a Day Are Dangerous

Many assume that smoking only a few cigarettes a day may not be dangerous. But studies have found that even very light smoking (as few as one to four cigarettes per day) can double the risk of heart attack in women. Some researchers have found an almost three times higher rate of heart attack in middle-aged men who smoked one to four cigarettes daily. Furthermore, no real benefit has been found in changing to low nicotine or "light" cigarettes as far as heart disease is concerned.

A Higher Risk in Those Who Don't Smoke

There is now ever increasing evidence that exposure to tobacco smoke *in persons who don't smoke cigarettes*—so-called second-hand smoke— increases their risk of heart attack. According to some researchers, this environmental tobacco smoke may result in up to 35,000 to 40,000 deaths each year due to coronary heart disease.

Stop Smoking and Reduce the Risk of Heart Attack

Studies show that the risk of coronary heart disease goes down dramatically when smoking is stopped. For example, the risk of coronary heart disease goes down by half after one year and continues to decrease with time. Estimates are that after five to fifteen years your risk is as low as if you never smoked cigarettes. For heart patients who quit smoking, the risk of a second heart attack also goes down quickly.

Studies reveal that among women who stopped cigarettes, the higher risk of heart attack dropped by one third after two years, and after ten to fourteen years the risk lowered to the level of nonsmokers. Other research has shown that the risk of heart attack increases by seven times in women who smoke fifteen to twenty-four cigarettes daily. Researchers have found that women who began smoking before age fifteen had over nine times the risk of coronary heart disease. Women who smoked and used oral birth control pills had a risk about twenty-three times higher for heart attack when they smoked more than twenty-five cigarettes per day.

Heart Risk from Smoking: Greatly Increased

A report of the Smoking Education Program of the National Institute of Health reviewed some of the areas of increased risk caused by smoking:

- coronary heart disease, especially heart attack and heart failure

- increased risk for coronary heart disease in those who already are at high risk due to hypertension and high blood cholesterol

- atherosclerosis and blockage of the arteries that supply the feet and legs—leading to gangrene and amputation

- atherosclerosis and blockage of the arteries that supply blood to the brain—leading to stroke

- increased risk of sudden death

- coronary heart disease and stroke in women who take oral contraceptives (especially after age thirty-five)

- increased blood cholesterol due to heightened LDL cholesterol and possible lowering of the HDL cholesterol

- impaired physical performance, endurance, and lung function.

Diabetes and Smoking

If you are diabetic, then you already run about twice the risk of heart disease. If you are diabetic *and* smoke cigarettes, the risk of heart disease increases another four to six times the normal rate. Although smoking is no more common among diabetics than others, there is greater danger of heart disease because of the already higher risk.

You Can *Kick the Habit*

Even though smoking increases the risk of heart attack, it is one risk factor that can be controlled. Make a commitment today to stop. If you have trouble stopping, talk to your doctor, or call your local chapter of the American Lung Association or American Cancer Society.

You may feel withdrawal symptoms for the first one to two weeks after you have stopped smoking, especially if you have been a heavy smoker. Nicotine patches (prescribed by your doctor) that are worn on the skin, nicotine gum or other medications can help you through the difficult initial period of withdrawal. Then the physical problem should be less troublesome, but the urge to smoke can always return. It is a matter of mental self-control, and you still may need the support of a spouse or friend.

Smoking cigarettes may be the one risk factor for heart attack that is most preventable. If you don't have heart disease, consider kicking the habit to lower your risk. If you already suffer from coronary heart disease, you have no choice: you *must* stop smoking to lower the risk of future heart attacks.

4. Diet

The amount and kind of food we eat can directly affect our bodies and thus prevent or contribute to disease. In fact, diet plays a major role in the risk of heart attack and coronary heart disease (see chapter 6 for a heart-healthy diet). There are at least two different ways diet can be important: the *type of foods* in your diet can reduce or raise your risk of heart disease. Also, if you are overweight, you can use diet to lower your risk of heart attack by *losing extra pounds*. Let's look at some examples of how certain foods can make a difference in the rate of heart attack.

Total Amount and Type of Fat Matter

The amount and the type of fat in your diet can make a major difference in your own risk of heart attack and coronary heart disease. For example, diets high in saturated fats (from animal tissue) often produce high blood cholesterol and therefore a higher risk of heart attack (see table 2.7).

But simply lowering the amount of fat in your diet may not help! In most cases, it is not just the *total* amount of fat in the diet that decides your risk of heart attack. For example, it has been found that over the past twenty years, even though the rate of heart attack has decreased, the total dietary fat for Americans has changed only a little. However, the total average cholesterol in the American diet has dropped from 700 to about 380 mg per day.

It would be a good idea to choose a diet that adjusts the *type* of fat, not merely the amount of fat in your diet. Basically, this means a diet with lower saturated fats and higher amounts of certain poly-unsaturated and monounsaturated fats (see p. 116). Ways of achieving this would be to use olive oil and polyunsaturated margarine; eat fish and lean meat; use skim milk (or 1–2 percent fat milk); and eat fresh fruit, vegetables, and more fiber. Meat can be a part of this diet! See chapter 7 for creative and easy-to-make diet choices.

Table 2.7
Foods High in Saturated Fats

Fast Foods	*Supermarket / Deli Foods*
Cheeseburger	Bacon
Donuts	Bologna
Egg-sausage sandwich	Many cheeses
French fries	Coconut
Fried chicken sandwich	Cream
Hot dog	Ground beef
Onion rings	Ham
Taco salad	Salami
	Sausage
	Sour cream
	Whipped cream

Examples of some fast food choices near or below the 30 percent-or-less fat guideline include: tossed green salads at most franchises (but choose a low-fat or vinegar and oil dressing); Burger King BK Broiler Chicken Sandwich (32 percent fat); McDonald's McGrilled Chicken Sandwich (28 percent fat); McDonald's frozen yogurt (0 percent fat); Wendy's baked potato with cheese and broccoli (27 percent fat); and Subway roast turkey breast sandwich (23 percent fat).

The Vegetarian Diet

Vegetarians (those who eat meat or poultry less than once each week) often have lower blood cholesterol levels than nonvegetarians. There are other factors involved, since vegetarians also often have other differences in their lifestyle. Some researchers have found that those who ate red meat or poultry less than once a week did in fact also engage in more physical activity. They were also less overweight and had lower cholesterol and triglyceride blood test results. These other lifestyle practices have an effect on their overall risk of heart attack.

However, only a small percentage of the entire population, mostly young adults, follows a vegetarian diet. Perhaps it is simply habit or most people find the pleasure of eating meat simply cannot be satisfied by such a restricted diet. In any case, you don't have to eliminate meat from the diet in order to control cholesterol.

The Mediterranean Diet

The "Mediterranean diet" is so called because it is common in some Southern European, North African, and Middle Eastern countries, which have a lower rate of heart attack. This diet includes the use of olive oil in place of other fat. Even though there may be surprisingly high overall fat intake, the amount of saturated fat eaten—contained in food such as meat and animal and dairy fats—is lower than in other countries.

Olive oil, cereals, pasta, legumes, fruit, fresh vegetables, and wine are also common to the Mediterranean diet. Certain fish, such as sardines and anchovies, are also common. Men who ate a diet rich in cereals, vegetables, fruit, fish, and olive oil had one-third the death rate from heart disease compared to those living in countries with high saturated fats in their diets.

What about Wine?

In France, where there is a *high* intake of saturated fat, including cholesterol from dairy fats and animal fats, surprisingly there is also a *low* death rate from heart attack and coronary heart disease. How can this be? Some researchers think that it may be due to the amount of wine consumed, often with meals.

Some recent studies have shown that those who drink the equivalent of one to two drinks per day seem to have fewer heart attacks than those who do not drink at all or those who have four or more drinks per day. (One drink constitutes about 12 ounces of beer, 5 ounces of wine, or 1.5 ounces of 80 proof distilled alcohol.) In Italy, the lowest risk for heart attack and cardiovascular disease was found in men who drank less than half a liter of wine per day. The exact reason is not known, but it may be that wine raises the HDL (the "good") cholesterol and may therefore give protection from coronary heart disease. Or alcohol may offer some protection against blood clotting in the coronary arteries.

Is wine more effective than other types of alcoholic drinks? Some studies, especially from the United States, suggest that beer, wine, and spirits are about equally protective in heart disease. Other evidence, especially from European studies, suggests that wine may actually be more protective than other types of alcohol. Or it may be that when wine is taken with meals it is absorbed slowly and gives a longer protective effect in the blood to prevent clotting. Some researchers believe that red wine may be more effective than white.

Experts have concluded that moderate amounts of alcohol (equal to about one to two drinks per day) may decrease the risk of heart attack by up to 40 percent. But be aware that if you do drink higher levels of alcohol, you can *increase* your risk of heart disease as well as other medical problems, such as liver disease.

The potential for harm has prevented a recommendation for everyone to drink alcohol to prevent heart attack. For example, pregnant women, those with liver disease or who are taking medications, and recovering alcoholics may increase their danger by adding alcohol. Since every person is different, you should talk to your doctor before you increase your alcohol intake to see what is best for you.

Certain Nuts Can Prevent Heart Attack

A recent study found that those who eat nuts more than four times weekly had fewer heart attacks and fewer deaths from heart attacks. This was true in both vegetarians and nonvegetarians. The nuts eaten were mainly peanuts, almonds, and walnuts. The causes of the protective effect are not known. Most of the calories in nuts come from fat, but there is a relatively high amount of polyunsaturated fat present which has a desirable effect on blood cholesterol. Also, linoleic acid is found in these nuts, which is a source of omega-6 polyunsaturated fat. Omega-6 and omega-3 polyunsaturated fatty acids may have a protective effect against heart disease.

Vitamin E

Vitamin E is not new, but many new facts about it have been discovered over the past few years. One of its jobs in the body is to remove oxidants created by normal chemical reactions in the body. Oxidants may have a part in the first minor injury to the inside walls of the arteries in coronary heart disease (discussed on p. 4). They may also make it easier for cholesterol deposits to enter the walls of arteries, which means that atherosclerosis may progress more quickly. Oxidants are removed by antioxidants which might slow down the process of atherosclerosis, with less blockage and fewer heart attacks.

Vitamin E, vitamin C, and beta carotene are natural antioxidants. Researchers have shown that men and women who took vitamin E supplements (at least 100 IU daily) had 25 to 50 percent less coronary heart disease.

No serious side effects from taking this amount of supplemental vitamin E are known, but longer term studies are in progress now. The amount of vitamin E taken in the above studies would require a specific supplement available at your pharmacy, grocery, or health food store. Natural sources of vitamin E, such as wheat germ oil and sunflower seeds, have low amounts of the vitamin.

Fiber

Fiber in the diet might also have a beneficial effect on heart attack. Some researchers have found that men who ate large amounts of bread and other cereal products had lower amounts of coronary heart disease. Whole grain cereal, oats, and other dietary fiber may lower your cholesterol level, especially if it is abnormally high. But so far, the evidence does not prove that fiber is an effective way to lower the risk of heart attack.

Coffee

There have been conflicting reports about whether drinking coffee raises the risk of heart attack. Some people smoke cigarettes when they drink coffee, which can confuse the results. Overall, the balance of evidence from most studies is that drinking coffee does *not* cause coronary heart disease and that at least as many as four cups a day does not increase the risk of heart attack.

For More on a Heart-Healthy Diet

Chapter 7 offers specific suggestions on how to be sure your diet gives you the best protection against heart attack, including the American Heart Association recommendations for a heart-healthy, low-fat diet and the use of antioxidants such as vitamin E.

5. Lack of regular exercise

The more regular your physical exercise, the lower your chance of heart attack and coronary heart disease. For those who have suffered a heart attack, studies have found increased risk of another attack at an earlier age and greater danger of death if they do little exercise. Researchers now agree that regular physical activity is an important part of the overall program to prevent heart attack.

Exercise and Prevention

Many researchers have shown that the greater your degree of physical fitness, the lower your risk of heart attack. This may be especially true for those who smoke cigarettes, suffer from hypertension, or have high blood cholesterol. Some studies have shown up to five times less risk for heart attack among those who were more fit. One long-term study of college alumni found that the rate of death from first heart attacks decreased as exercise from walking, climbing stairs, and sports activity increased.

Regular Exercise Helps Cholesterol

Regular physical exercise lowers the levels of cholesterol and LDL cholesterol, which in turn reduces the risk of heart attack. Exercise also raises the HDL cholesterol, which also helps protect against heart attack. Some experts estimate that walking even about eight to ten miles per week may be enough to raise the HDL cholesterol. One study showed that middle-aged women who exercised were better able to maintain weight control and retain higher levels of HDL cholesterol with its protective effect.

Exercise Helps Blood Pressure

A regular exercise program can also lower blood pressure, often by about 10 mm Hg., which can reduce the risk of heart attack. And exercise can help decrease stress, which also lowers your heart attack risk. Some researchers have found that those who had better fitness also were less overweight, less hypertensive, and had better overall cholesterol levels.

Exercise Makes the Heart Efficient

With exercise training, the pumping action of the heart can become more efficient. Coronary artery blood flow may even improve in some patients after supervised cardiac rehabilitation exercise programs. Some studies show that those patients who were given a cardiac rehabilitation exercise program after heart attack had 20 to 25 percent lower rate of fatal heart attacks thereafter.

Evidence suggests that the improvement in ability to exercise in those with coronary heart disease can occur with short periods of exercise (e.g., a ten-minute session three times daily). The improvement was similar to that from one daily 30-minute session. Walking, even slowly, is probably the easiest exercise to follow and to control. Walking even less than two miles per hour may be enough to cause improvement at first. Ask your doctor how much and how fast you should walk.

There are fewer specific studies of cardiac rehabilitation in women than in men. However, the evidence is that the same improvement can occur in women with cardiac rehabilitation and exercise after heart attack, even though they may more often suffer from hypertension, diabetes, and higher blood cholesterol. Many women may improve as much as or more than men in ability to exercise after a three-month program.

Patients Who Are Winning with Exercise

Carolyn D., a 60-year-old beauty shop owner, had her first heart attack at age fifty-eight. "I should have known this would happen," she said, "because of our family history. Both of my parents had heart attacks at an early age."

Carolyn should have also taken precautions to reduce her risk factors. "I smoked, ate anything that tasted good, and never exercised," she told us. "After the heart attack, my doctor suggested that I stop cigarettes immediately, then begin exercise to reduce my stress and risk factors for further heart problems. I started to walk—only around the block at first. I was huffing and puffing; I thought I would die just doing that short walk! But I was determined that I would do this. I walked every evening, then again in the morning. In one month, I had stopped smoking and was walking one and a half miles."

When Carolyn was seen three months after her heart attack, she had changed her diet using the heart-healthy recommendations in chapter 7, had quit smoking, and was walking three miles every evening after work. Her blood pressure was normal, her breathing clear, and her energy improved.

Another heart attack patient, Rick W., found that exercise saved his life. "After my heart attack, I made up my mind to start exercising," he told us. "I always knew that I should, but it was so much trouble. If you ever have the pain and fear of heart attack you will know to go to the trouble *before* it happens."

Rick started slowly on an exercise plan and is now walking four miles a day, three times a week. On his "off" days, Rick plays golf or tennis, or swims. "I do something each day for me," he said. "I want to beat this monster called heart attack."

Training Lowers Risk

Studies have shown that with a regular training program, heart attack patients run a lower risk of later death from heart disease. Coronary bypass patients can help maintain bypassed arteries with a regular training program. After heart attack only your doctor can decide what amount of exercise is best for you, as discussed on pp. 107ff. Many patients become much more active *after* a heart attack than they were before as a result of the planned exercise program.

How Much Exercise Is Enough?

A low to moderate level of exercise can achieve a good level of fitness. Of course, you should always check with your doctor before you start any exercise program since you may have some special needs or restrictions. It may be a good idea to have an exercise electrocardiogram before beginning, especially if you have not been very active. It is most important that you start slowly—but plan to *stay with it* and gradually increase your level of activity.

For prevention of heart attack, some types of exercise programs that are easy to carry out at home include: walking, bicycling (or exercise bike), swimming, and aerobic dancing and exercises. Choose one or more types of exercise convenient for your lifestyle and ones that you don't mind doing. If you hate the exercise, you probably won't keep it up for very long.

Some forms of exercise are better for very busy people. An exercise bike or treadmill at home, for example, can be used twenty-four hours a day with no excuses for bad weather. Jumping rope, jogging, and swimming are all ways to achieve excellent exercise in a brief workout. The goal could be to exercise fifteen to twenty minutes every day, five days a week. The amount of exercise needed after a heart attack is discussed on p. 108. Remember, exercise *can* help:

- lower LDL cholesterol and raise HDL cholesterol

- lower blood pressure

- lower stress

- control weight

- lower the risk of future heart attacks.

What about Strength Training?

Can weight lifting and similar exercises help? The problem with weight lifting is that it often causes a greater increase in blood pressure and heart rate than some of the above exercises. For heart patients, this could be dangerous; however, a program of light weights or isometric exercises may be prescribed by your physician at certain times. You should definitely talk to your doctor before beginning any program using weights or isometric exercises.

Getting Started

When you begin an exercise program, begin slowly and gradually increase. For example, walk for two to three minutes, then gradually increase so that you don't feel tired or out of breath when you finish. You will be surprised at how quickly you can increase up to one to two miles daily. The most important goal is to keep up the program. The benefits happen when the program is long-lasting over months and years.

The American College of Sports Medicine recommends a goal of about fifteen to sixty minutes of vigorous exercise done three to five times each week. Studies offer evidence that this amount of exercise can increase cardiovascular fitness and will probably provide some protection against coronary heart disease. Exercise on the job may also be beneficial, but its effects are harder to prove. Lower levels of exercise may help, but are also not yet proven to be beneficial.

Make It Easy

You don't always have to exercise in one session each day. As we've said, three ten-minute sessions of walking probably give as much benefit as one thirty-minute session. This may allow your exercise to be more convenient with less fatigue.

Walking briskly, starting slowly and gradually working up to four to five miles per hour with arms swinging will provide the amount of exercise needed (discussed below). Holding light handweights while you walk ("power walking") can also be added as your fitness improves. If you feel short of breath or have any chest discomfort, then, of course, you should stop immediately and talk to your doctor before continuing.

Exercise after Heart Attack

If you have already had a heart attack or have coronary heart disease, your doctor must tell you how to begin an exercise program. It may be a good idea for your progress to be monitored in a cardiac rehabilitation exercise program which can allow close supervision of your exercise to ensure there are no irregular heartbeats, chest pains, shortness of breath, or other problems.

Experts consider exercise safe for most patients after heart attack or coronary artery surgery. Each person should have a carefully planned prescription for exercise to gain the most benefit while maintaining maximum safety. The chances of heart attack, cardiac arrest, or sudden death during exercise in cardiac rehabilitation are very low. If your doctor decides that you are at higher risk for problems, you can be monitored with an electrocardiogram while you exercise.

Minor Injuries Can Happen

You may have minor injuries such as sprains, strains and pain when you exercise, especially from overuse injuries (such as doing too much exercise at first or increasing the level of exercise to quickly). These are usually short-term injuries that may slow you down or make you stop exercising temporarily.

6. Being Overweight

There are many jokes about overweight people, but in fact it is no laughing matter. Hypertension and diabetes mellitus are three times more likely in obese persons. Obesity also increases the risk of cancer of the colon, rectum, and prostate in men. In women, obesity increases the risk of cancer of the breast, uterus, and ovaries, and gall bladder. It is important to plan to lose your excess pounds. You don't have to become slim, but losing enough weight to lower your risk of heart attack is a very good goal.

A person is overweight if his or her body weight is 20 percent or more above desirable weight (see table 2.8). National surveys have found that 24 percent of men and 27 percent of women are overweight using this measure; for example, a man of "average" height of 5'9" who weighs over 187 pounds or an "average" woman of 5'4" who weighs over 158 pounds is considered overweight.

Hypertension Increases with Excess Weight

The more overweight you are, the higher your risk for hypertension: one estimate showed almost three times the risk for hypertension. LDL (the "bad") cholesterol and triglyceride levels are often higher in overweight people, while HDL cholesterol levels are often lower. These changes in blood cholesterol and triglycerides can increase the risk of coronary heart disease. Being overweight also increases the risk of diabetes mellitus, which itself increases the danger of heart disease, as discussed on p. 47. The way in which excess weight causes hypertension and high blood cholesterol may be due to changes in the way the body handles the hormone insulin.

Overweight persons have a higher risk of heart attack. In fact, the more overweight, the higher the chance of death from heart attack as well as other causes.

Waist and Hip Measurement Matters!

If you are overweight, the strongest risk for heart disease is when the excess weight and fat is concentrated in the abdomen—an increase in *waist* size compared to the hips—not simply overall fat distribution. Researchers recommend that the ratio of the waist size to the hip size in men be 1:1 or less and in women 0.8:1. For example, a man whose waist size is 36 inches should have a hip size of about 36 inches. And a woman whose waist size is 28 inches should have a hip size of about 35 inches.

Table 2.8
1983 Metropolitan Height and Weight Table

Men

Height				
Feet	*Inches*	*Small Frame*	*Medium Frame*	*Large Frame*
5	2	128–134	131–141	138–150
5	3	130–136	133–143	140–153
5	4	132–138	135–145	142–156
5	5	134–140	137–148	144–160
5	6	136–142	139–151	146–164
5	7	138–145	142–154	149–168
5	8	140–148	145–157	152–172
5	9	142–151	148–160	155–176
5	10	144–154	151–163	158–180
5	11	146–157	154–166	161–184
6	0	149–160	157–170	164–188
6	1	152–164	160–174	168–192
6	2	155–168	164–178	172–197
6	3	158–172	167–182	176–202
6	4	162–176	171–187	181–207

Check Your Weight

Check your proper body weight in table 2.8 to see where you fit in.
If you weigh more than 20 percent beyond your ideal body weight,
make your commitment to begin a weight loss program. Easy steps
you can take to lose weight for good—painlessly and without starvation—
are discussed in chapter 7. Talk to your doctor for advice.

7. Stress

Stress and the way you manage it may play an important part in your
risk of heart attack. It is a very common belief that high stress may
contribute to heart attacks. One large survey of men asked whether
they felt tension, anxiety or difficulty sleeping from conditions at work
or at home. The men who felt higher degrees of stress were also found
to develop more coronary heart disease.

Table 2.8
1983 Metropolitan Height and Weight Table (cont'd.)

Women

Height		Small Frame	Medium Frame	Large Frame
Feet	*Inches*			
4	10	102–111	109–121	118–131
4	11	103–113	111–123	120–134
5	0	104–115	113–126	122–137
5	1	106–118	115–129	125–140
5	2	108–121	118–132	128–143
5	3	111–124	121–135	131–147
5	4	114–127	124–138	134–151
5	5	117–130	127–141	137–155
5	6	120–133	130–144	140–159
5	7	123–136	133–147	143–163
5	8	126–139	136–150	146–167
5	9	129–142	139–153	149–170
5	10	132–145	142–156	152–173
5	11	135–148	145–159	155–176
6	0	138–151	148–162	158–179

Weights at ages 25–59 based on lowest mortality. Weight in pounds according to fram (in indoor clothing weighing 3 lbs. for women, 5 lbs. for men, shoes with 1″ heels).

Source: 1979 Build Study, Society of Actuaries and Association of Life Insurance Medical Directors of America, 1980. Reprinted courtesy Metropolitan Life Insurance Company.

Stress is normal and not necessarily a bad thing; it can lead us into actions to solve problems. For example, if we feel stress from finding an abnormal blood pressure and take action to make it normal, the stress has been very useful. But stress of many types can also contribute to hypertension, excess eating, and limited exercise as a result of fatigue. These added problems can also contribute to increased risk of heart attack.

Emotional stress can increase blood pressure and heart rate, which increases the workload on the heart. Stressful, emotional events in our lives, such as the death of a family member, a divorce, or the loss of a job can cause stress on the heart and even trigger heart attack. One survey of heart attack patients found three times as many deaths in those who had high stress levels that were left untreated. Remember the saying used in stressful situations, "Don't have a heart attack."

Some jobs are more stressful and demanding than others. For example, driving a bus in a large city is known to be very stressful. In fact, there is a higher risk of hypertension, heart disease, and death among city bus drivers in many different countries. The exact connection between this kind of stress and heart attack is not known.

Psychological stress has also been found in workers whose jobs are excessively demanding but allow little influence in managing those demands. Workers who have fewer demands, more manageable demands, and who also have good social support have a lower risk of heart disease.

If you feel your own stress is reaching an uncomfortable level, consider getting advice on stress management from a clinical psychologist or psychiatrist. Techniques can be easily learned to control stress and anxiety and lower your risk of heart attack. These are successful, and are commonly taught to heart attack patients. Adjustments in these traits can be life-saving by lowering the risk of future heart attacks.

Some easy steps to help control anxiety and stress are discussed in chapter 8.

8. Personality and Behavior

Personality and behavior may play a role in heart disease. For example, the Type A personality denotes a hard-driving, competitive and aggressive temperament. These persons may be impatient, very competitive, anxious to accomplish several tasks, strongly motivated toward achievement, and full of aggression and hostility that they often keep inside. How do you fit in?

Are You a Type A or B Personality?

The following characteristics are common among those with type A personality. The more of them you have, the more likely you are to be a type A personality.

- I am usually hard-driving and competitive.

- I usually feel pressed for time.

- I am often bossy and demanding.

- I have a strong need to be the best in most things.

- I often feel pressed for time at the end of the working day.

- I often get upset or angry when I have to wait for something or someone doesn't agree with me.

Hostility and Anger

The specific parts of the Type A personality that seem to bring with them the greatest risk for heart attack are *hostility* and *anger*. It is not known why these specific traits cause heart attacks. However, they often do cause an increase in feelings of stress and anxiety, which effect the changes in heart rate and blood pressure discussed earlier. Some researchers also have found higher cholesterol in the diets of those with greater levels of hostility!

Persons with Type B personalities, on the other hand, are often more relaxed, easy going, and less hurried; therefore, they may have a lower risk of heart attack. Type B personality may allow for a better sense of inner security without as much need to compete and with less fear of failure. These people accomplish at the same level as Type A personalities, but with much less stress and heart risk.

9. Sex and Menopause

Men are at higher risk of heart attack than women until women reach the age of menopause. The increased risk of heart attack among post-menopausal women is thought to be due to the loss of the female hormone estrogen.

Before menopause, women usually have lower LDL cholesterol and higher HDL cholesterol than men. After menopause, as estrogen levels become lower, the HDL cholesterol level goes down and LDL cholesterol level goes up. Both these changes in the body's cholesterol raise the risk of heart attack.

Estrogen treatment after menopause decreases LDL cholesterol and increases HDL cholesterol, thus protecting against heart attack. If progestin hormones are also added after menopause, there may be less improvement in HDL cholesterol from estrogen.

Less Heart Disease with Estrogen after Menopause

Studies of women show less heart disease when estrogen is given after menopause. Women who take estrogen have about a 40 to 50 percent lesser chance of heart attack and other coronary heart disease than those who don't. Estrogen also protects against other cardiovascular diseases. This occurs through an increase in HDL cholesterol.

While estrogen pills are shown to produce this positive effect, estrogen given by injection or patch has a less predictable effect in reducing cholesterol.

Estrogen's Side Effects

Possible side effects of taking estrogen treatment after menopause include a slightly higher risk of uterine cancer, which can be controlled if there is regular followup with your doctor. A simple test can be done in the office to detect the uterine cancer very early and at a stage when it can be easily treated. Talk with your doctor.

There is also a slightly increased risk of breast cancer in certain women who take estrogen after menopause. Those who have had breast cancer or breast cysts or a family history of breast cancer may be at a higher risk. Each person is different, so consult your doctor.

Other problems such as blood clots (thrombophlebitis) have been thought to occur more often when estrogen is used after menopause, although there is less evidence of this in recent studies.

Despite the good results obtained with estrogen treatment after menopause, this therapy is still not recommended for every woman. However, those at higher risk, such as those who already have coronary heart disease, high cholesterol, or other risk factors may well benefit. The overall benefits and risks must be taken into consideration by you as an individual when you talk with your doctor.

Should estrogen treatment be started even many years after the menopause? The best answer depends on studies now in progress, so you should discuss with your doctor what steps to take in your own case. The benefits should outweigh the potential risks when contemplating such therapy.

Birth Control Pills

Oral contraceptives (birth control pills) contain a combination of an estrogen and progesterone hormone. While the estrogen increases HDL cholesterol and lowers LDL cholesterol, the progestin part of the birth control pill tends to decrease HDL cholesterol and increase LDL cholesterol, which could increase the chance of heart disease.

Newer pills have improved combinations of the two medications and recent studies show no increased risk of heart disease with the newer combinations *if* the woman does not also smoke and has no other risk factors. As discussed on p. 30, the risk of heart attack is especially high if a woman smokes and takes oral birth control pills.

10. Age

The risk of heart attack and coronary heart disease increases with age, as do the levels of total cholesterol and LDL cholesterol. However, atherosclerosis can actually begin in childhood. Microscopic evidence of changes in the artery walls has been found even in children. By adolescence there may be visible streaks due to atherosclerosis in the wall of the arteries. Among people aged twenty to thirty, especially those with other risk factors, there may be further changes in the arteries.

In men the process gradually increases after age thirty. In women the increase begins later, after menopause, between the ages of forty-five and fifty-five. Coronary heart disease becomes more prominent in men after age forty and in women after age fifty, when it becomes the most common cause of death. After age sixty-five coronary heart disease gradually increases with age in both men and women.

11. Diabetes Mellitus

The chance of coronary heart disease and heart attack is increased two to six times in diabetics, and diabetes may pose an even stronger risk to women than men—twice the risk according to one study. Those who have suffered a heart attack run a higher risk of death if diabetes is present, although the exact reasons for this are not known.

Among women with diabetes who smoke, and are also hypertensive or overweight, the risk for heart attack is increased threefold. Some research has shown that diabetics who were treated without insulin more often had less HDL (the "good") cholesterol, were more overweight, and had higher triglyceride levels. Each of these factors raises the risk to the heart. When the blood glucose in diabetes is not well controlled, the levels of triglycerides and cholesterol may be higher, thus posing additional risk of heart attack.

A blood test is the best way to discover diabetes mellitus, and is

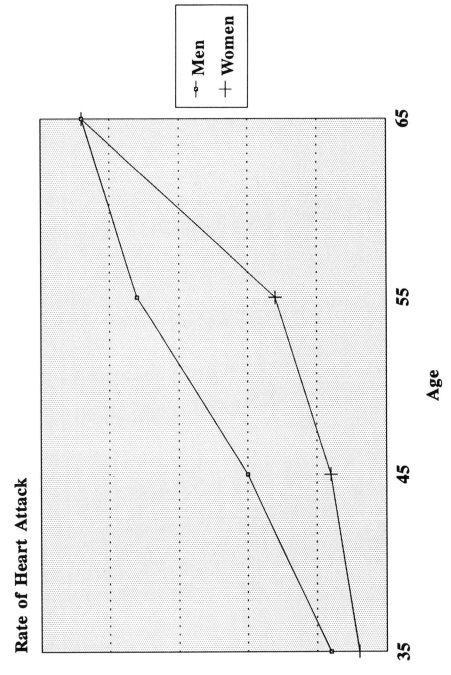

Figure 2.3
The risk of heart attack increases with age.

part of many routine examinations. If your blood glucose is abnormal, be sure to talk with your doctor and make a plan. Begin diet, weight control and medication if needed to maintainthe best possible control of your blood glucose. Control the other risk factors to lower your risk of heart attack to the lowest level.

12. Family History

You may be at higher risk for heart attack if you have a male family member under age fifty-five or a female family member under age sixty-five who had a heart attack or other coronary heart disease. While this is a risk factor that cannot be removed, there may be ways to manage it. In many cases, the family member affected by heart disease also suffers from hypertension or high blood cholesterol, or smokes. These risk factors *can* be controlled to lower your own risk. If you have a family history of early coronary heart disease, then take extra effort to detect and control your own risk factors as early as possible.

The problem is, in part, genetic. Genes passed from parents to offspring control the way our bodies work. Some genes control the way in which the body manages fats such as cholesterol, including LDL and HDL cholesterol. These in turn directly affect the rate of atherosclerosis and heart attack. If you are genetically predisposed to high blood cholesterol, you will then inherit a higher risk of heart attack. In fact, it may be a combination of genes and such risk factors as hypertension, cigarette smoking, diet, and exercise that actually result in heart attack.

In the future, there may be ways to correct the actions of the genes— until then you can check your other risk factors to control your risk of heart disease.

YOU *CAN* WIN!

It is possible to win with heart attack today. Research has shown ways to eliminate important risk factors, such as controlling your diet to reduce cholesterol, exercising to reduce hypertension, or kicking the smoking habit. But all the research in the world won't make a difference until every person becomes responsible for his or her well-being and lifestyle.

Are you doing all you can to eliminate your risk factors for heart attack? Check your personal risk factors using the form on p. 51. The facts do not lie regarding your personal risks. But the good news is that many of these components can be changed! Write down some attainable goals that will help you gain control of your health, and start a program today to get in shape. You and your heart will be glad you did!

Personal Risk Factor Assessment

Name _____

Date _____

1. Sex: Male —— Female ——

2. Age: _____ .

3. Height and weight: _____'_____" and _____ lbs.
   Ideal weight from pp. 42–43: _____

4. Blood pressure reading: _____ . Date _____ .

5. Total cholesterol: _____ . LDL cholesterol: _____ .
   HDL cholesterol: _____ . Triglycerides: _____ .

6. Smoking: (circle) Yes No

7. Low-fat diet: (circle) Yes No

8. Use of polyunsaturated and monounsaturated fats: Yes No

9. Regular exercise: Low Moderate High

10. Rate your stress: Low Moderate High

11. Type A or B Personality: (circle) A B

12. (If female) postmenopausal: Yes No
    Estrogen treatment: Yes No

13. Diabetes: Yes No

14. Family history of heart attack: Father's age _____
                                    Mother's age _____
                                    Sibling's age _____

Personal Goal Setting

On this page, write down those factors you need to eliminate or control and how you will do this. For example, if you do little exercise, begin a walking program, working up to two miles, four times a week. If your diet is high in fat, check chapter 7, purchase a heart-healthy cookbook, and relearn the way you eat, focusing on a diet higher in fruits and vegetables, and low in saturated fats. Take control of your health and your risk factors!

Name _____

Date _____

1.

2.

3.

4.

5.

6.

7.

8.

9.

10.

3

Signs and Symptoms

Most of us are familiar with some classic symptoms of heart attack—severe chest pain, pain traveling down the left arm, shortness of breath. But did you know that you can have heart attack without any unusual feelings at all? Do you know which symptoms need evaluation? It is important to understand all the feelings or signs that can warn about coronary heart disease or heart attack. If treatment is given at the earliest stages, you have the best chance of survival without damage and the best chance of living a normal, active life.

Remember, the more risk factors you have, the higher the chances are that you might develop coronary heart disease. Being aware of the fact that a heart attack could happen to *you* is important to your long-term health. Early detection is also important if you develop heart disease, since many of the complications can be prevented with treatment.

COMMON SIGNS OF HEART ATTACK

The most common initial feeling or sign of coronary heart disease is discomfort in the chest. This can be a sensation of *tightness, pressure, dull pain, squeezing, heaviness, aching, indigestion, burning or other discomfort, or a combination of any of these.* It can happen at rest or may occur only with some exertion such as walking, working, lifting, or after a large meal. This might even come on when you are not active, especially at night, and it may awaken you from sleep. Some notice these feelings first during a sudden change in activity such as shoveling snow after the first snowstorm.

The chest pain or discomfort may move around and might be felt in the *shoulder, arm, neck, jaw, or back.* At times, there may only be discomfort in the shoulder or arm, with little or no pain in the chest.

There may be *shortness of breath,* which is usually mild. This usually disappears along with the chest discomfort. Some persons also experience *sweating or nausea.* This might come on when you are not active, especially at first, or the sweating and nausea might awaken you from sleep.

DON'T OVERLOOK THE SYMPTOMS

In some cases it will be easy to overlook or ignore the feelings. You may have only arm or jaw pain, or the feeling might be dismissed as merely indigestion.

When any chest discomfort above as described is caused by coronary heart disease, it is called *angina pectoris,* Latin for chest pain. The feelings usually last only a few minutes and relief normally comes from sitting and resting for a few minutes or by taking nitroglycerin medication. At times the activity causing the pain can be predicted and avoided. For instance, some persons find that angina comes on only if they are walking too fast, walking uphill, or in cold weather. Some notice it only if they do all three.

Of concern is the fact that at times, even though there is a serious problem, *there may be no feeling of chest pain or discomfort at all. This is called "silent" ischemia* or "silent" angina pectoris.* It is very common and certainly as serious as when there is chest discomfort. Silent ischemia can be detected by special testing, as discussed in chapter 4.

Table 3.1
Common Symptoms of Heart Attack

- A feeling in the chest such as:
    tightness
    pressure
    dull pain
    squeezing
    heaviness
    aching
    indigestion
    burning
    other discomfort or a combination of any of these.

---

*Ischemia occurs when there is an inadequate supply of blood and oxygen to the heart muscle.

Table 3.1 (cont'd.)

- Pain felt in:
  shoulder
  arm
  neck
  jaw
  back

- Shortness of breath

- Nausea and sweating.

BE SMART! SEE YOUR DOCTOR

Any of the above signs or symptoms should alert you to talk to your doctor. If it is the first time the feeling occurs or if it lasts for more than a few minutes, then call your doctor immediately. If you know you have coronary heart disease, and the discomfort lasts longer than usual or comes on more often than usual, you should call your doctor or immediately pick up the telephone and dial 911.

If you ignore these feelings, you may be at risk of a heart attack. Heart attacks have a 50 percent death rate if they happen outside of the hospital, usually as a result of very irregular heart beats (arrhythmia) which can be treated if discovered in a hospital; the irregular rhythm cannot be effectively treated at home.

Don't give in to a common temptation to ignore or deny these feelings—check them out with your doctor. Don't be embarrassed to describe what may seem like trivial or meaningless signs or feelings. *These may be the only warning signs of serious coronary heart disease you will ever have!*

Simon R. is a 52-year-old man who noticed that during golf he experienced chest tightness when walking up a hill: "I had this experience three or four times on the golf course over one month," Simon said. "I honestly thought they would go away and ignored them, but at the time of my routine checkup, I decided I better talk about it with my doctor."

Simon had tests which eventually revealed blockage of a major degree in one coronary artery, while the others showed little change. Following successful angioplasty with a balloon-tipped catheter, Simon has returned to golf without any limits.

If Simon had continued to ignore the discomfort, he might have had far more serious problems with a heart attack. This would have meant much more time out of work recovering, and increased expense. Simon was smart to save time and suffering by taking steps early when treatment is most effective.

Mark H. was forty years old when he felt chest discomfort. "It was not horrible or burning," he told us. "But when I mowed the lawn last Saturday, I had a tightness in my chest that I could not explain."

Mark may not seem like a prime candidate for heart attack because of his age, but we heard his description of chest discomfort and his family history, with his father and uncle both having had heart attacks before age forty-five. Further tests also showed a blockage in one coronary artery. Like Simon, Mark had successful angioplasty with a balloon-tipped catheter, and is now as active as ever.

ANY CHEST DISCOMFORT NEEDS ATTENTION

Even if you have *none* of the risk factors discussed in chapter 2, do not hesitate to call your doctor if you have chest discomfort. It is too important to overlook this problem when early treatment is most effective. If you have any question and you are unsure what to do, call your doctor or go to an emergency room for evaluation. Don't ever be too embarrassed to seek treatment.

One patient, Sylvia M., had been experiencing chest pains for several days before she finally called her doctor. "I did not want to cry wolf," she told us. "My husband always says that I act hysterically, so I wanted to wait until I was sure it was my heart."

Don't *ever* wait to do this! The earlier you seek care, the more effective the treatment is likely to be. Excellent treatment is available (see chapter 5) after the diagnosis is made.

TYPES OF ANGINA PECTORIS

Stable Angina Pectoris

Stable angina pectoris means that the discomfort and limitation have not increased recently, such as over the last one to two months. There may be chest pain, tightness or other discomfort on exertion or from other causes, but the severity and frequency of the episodes is the same. The chest discomfort usually lasts less than five minutes and is relieved by resting or by nitroglycerin medication.

In persons with stable angina, researchers usually find a narrowing of at least one of the coronary arteries. The narrowed blood vessel allows enough blood (and oxygen) supply to the heart muscle at rest. With more activity, the heart increases its work and needs more blood, but the narrowed vessel limits the supply of blood and angina develops. With rest, the need for more blood supply lessens, and the chest pain goes away. Medication such as nitroglycerin may relieve the pain in a few minutes, and other medications can help prevent angina. Your doctor needs to direct your treatment.

Sandra W., sixty-five, had occasional chest tightness over one year, which she described as "a squeezing sensation under my breast bone." She told of the tightness lasting for two to three minutes. It happened almost exclusively if Sandra hurried when walking to her office, especially in cool weather. If she stopped walking or took a nitroglycerin spray, the tightness went away. Sandra had no other complaints or limitations.

Sandra was carefully monitored by her doctor, who did a few tests and prescribed a medication allowing her to follow all her usual daily activities without any real limits. She takes an aspirin each day, vitamin E supplements, and follows a low cholesterol diet.

Unstable Angina Pectoris

Angina pectoris is called unstable when the chest discomfort described above happens for the first time or when it becomes more frequent or longer lasting. This is important because it means danger, a higher risk of sudden worsening of the coronary heart disease at this time.

In unstable angina pectoris, chest discomfort may occur more often or with much less activity or exertion than before. It commonly happens with no activity at all—even awakening from sleep. Unstable angina pectoris can happen after a heart attack or in a patient who already has coronary heart disease, as discussed in chapter 5.

Susan O., a 70-year-old retired executive, had had stable angina pectoris for several years, but took medications and experienced only mild limitations. She walked three times each week for exercise and rarely had any chest discomfort. One day several months ago, Susan noticed a change: while she was walking, angina came on after only a few blocks, a distance she usually walked with no trouble. She called her doctor after she suffered an attack of angina while lying in bed.

Susan was admitted to the hospital; following tests to make sure no permanent heart damage was present, her medications were adjusted. Susan has resumed her usual activities after three months of a supervised exercise program at a cardiac rehabilitation outpatient center.

Unstable angina pectoris can happen suddenly with no specific cause, even when you have done everything as prescribed. Patients need immediate medical attention and hospitalization during any of the above types of unstable angina pectoris or prolonged chest pain.

Researchers have found that in unstable angina pectoris there is usually a sudden decrease in the blood flow in a coronary artery. This can happen from a small crack or fissure in the wall of the artery as discussed on p. 4. The fissure causes a reaction nearby, resulting in a clot in the artery and temporary blockage of the blood flow. The actual cause of the crack or fissure is not known.

PROLONGED CHEST PAIN

If chest discomfort lasts for more than twenty minutes then it is also treated as unstable angina pectoris, especially in a person who has had a heart attack or coronary artery surgery in the past. This is because there is now a higher risk of worsening, including heart attack with irregular heart beat and the risk of sudden death.

HEART ATTACK (MYOCARDIAL INFARCTION)

Any of the types of unstable angina pectoris just discussed can lead on to heart attack. Fortunately, most of the time unstable angina does not lead to actual death of heart muscle. But if the blood flow continues to be severely limited or stopped altogether for a long enough time, then there may be actual death of some of the heart muscle and a diagnosis of myocardial infarction.

It May Be the First Sign

Heart attack can happen without any warning signs at all. In up to one-third of all heart attacks, it is the first sign of coronary heart disease.

The chest discomfort may be sudden, severe and dramatic. Some describe the feeling as if "an elephant is sitting on my chest." Others tell of having the feeling of a "hot poker" through the chest. Still others have only mild tightness, pressure or indigestion. Any of the feelings described above for angina pectoris can occur in heart attack with the discomfort usually lasting more than a few minutes to several hours. It is dangerous to wait at home when these feelings occur. *This is the period of highest risk in heart attack.*

There May Be No Chest Pain

The chest discomfort may travel to one or both arms or to the neck or jaw. At times, there may be pain only in an arm or jaw with no noticeable chest pain. Dizziness may occur and the person affected may collapse, especially if the heart rhythm is irregular.

There is often shortness of breath with a feeling of suffocation. Sweating is common, and may even be the first sign. There may be nausea, vomiting or a feeling of the need to have a bowel movement.

Heart attacks can happen at any time of day or night, but are most common in morning hours, between 5 A.M. and noon. This happens to be when the blood pressure is commonly higher.

Most critical in the successful treatment of heart attack is timing. Since the first one to two hours are when most deaths happen in heart attack, it is extremely important to get medical attention quickly. *Call 911 or your local emergency medical service.* This is the time when patients commonly delay getting proper care: reasons range from denial of a problem to not wanting to trouble anyone. Many times a family member or friend helps make the decision to seek emergency care.

Lee A., fifty-nine, first noticed chest pain and tightness while walking up the ramp to a football game. The pain lasted a few minutes, but he really wanted to see the game. Lee ignored the pain, went to his seat, and collapsed about twenty minutes later. He was resuscitated by the quick action of an emergency medical team at the stadium and fortunately survived. Lee was found to have severe coronary artery disease and underwent coronary bypass surgery.

Bill P, forty-six, was at his son's soccer game when he noticed chest tightness that made him feel weak. He had been treated for heart disease several years earlier. He refused to allow a friend to call for help from emergency medical service, but the friend called anyway. Bill was found to have had a heart attack, and underwent tests that showed coronary blockage. He had successful angioplasty (see p. 77) and since has returned to work.

Yvonne C., sixty years old, had hypertension and smoked half a pack of cigarettes daily. She experienced quite severe indigestion during a Thanksgiving meal and found no relief with antacids. Yvonne thought she would rest and feel better later; however, after twenty minutes the indigestion grew worse and she broke out in a sweat. Her family insisted on taking her to the closest emergency room, where she was found to have had a heart attack! She suffered irregular heart beats which were treated and controlled. Yvonne was discharged following treatment and has since resumed her work as a professor. She stopped smoking and is working on other risk factor control.

DIAGNOSIS OF HEART ATTACK

The diagnosis of heart attack (myocardial infarction) is made after talking with the patient, an examination, an electrocardiogram (ECG or EKG), and other tests as discussed in chapter 4. Researchers have found that heart attack is usually the result of more complete blockage of blood flow after a crack or fissure in the thickened wall of an artery. A clot (thrombosis) forms at that site, which suddenly stops the blood flow (see figure 3.1).

The electrocardiogram is used to help diagnose myocardial infarction. There may be permanent ECG changes (called Q-wave infarction), which indicate a more complete and longer lasting blockage of the coronary artery and possibly death of heart muscle. In many cases, this is thought to be due to a larger crack or fissure in the wall of the artery, which causes a more severe clot.

In myocardial infarction there may be no permanent ECG changes (called non-Q-wave infarction). This is thought to be either because the blockage of the blood vessel did not last long enough or because other arteries made up for the loss of blood supply. In this type of myocardial infarction, there may be less actual permanent damage or death in the heart muscle itself. However, there is still risk in the future.

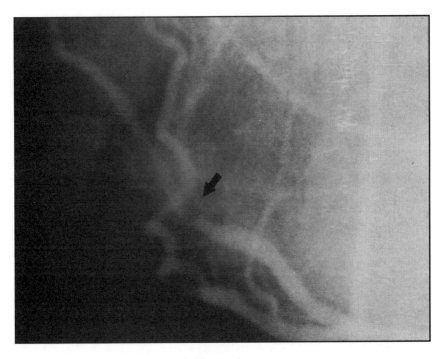

Figure 3.1
Heart attack results when the blood flow is blocked in a coronary artery.
The arrow shows the point of blockage.

SUDDEN CARDIAC DEATH

Unfortunately, death can occur suddenly in coronary heart disease. The most common cause is irregular heart beat (arrhythmia), which essentially stops the heart and its pumping action. In these cases there is usually a rapid and severe coronary artery clot and blockage of blood flow.

Researchers have found that 40 to 50 percent of those who have heart attacks may die. Up to 50 percent of those deaths occur in the first few hours, and up to 70 to 80 percent die in the first twenty-four hours, *mainly from the irregular heart beat.* The point is that the early hours are most dangerous because of the irregular heart beats—but these can be controlled once medical treatment is available. In the hospital, where good treatment is available for the irregular heart beats, the danger lessens.

DON'T IGNORE WARNINGS

If you have any of the feelings or signs discussed here, you should *contact your doctor immediately*. In many cases you may find that there are other explanations for your chest discomfort. For example, it is common to find problems, such as irritation of the esophagus (esophagitis), which cause indigestion and chest pain. Asthma or chronic bronchitis can result in shortness of breath and tightness in the chest. There are actually many different causes of chest discomfort which can mimic heart pain.

Simply talking to your doctor may offer you peace of mind about how likely it is that the pain is originating from the heart. If a few tests are needed to be sure, it is well worth it. The stakes are too high to ignore these feelings.

In the event that your problem is actually from coronary heart disease, you can then get early and effective treatment. The next steps in diagnosis, treatment, and prevention are discussed in chapters 4, 5, and 6. But by far the most important step is the one that you must take yourself—talk to your doctor or go to the nearest emergency treatment center.

4

Tests You May Need

When we saw 60-year-old Sam R. in the hospital, he had been having chest pains for more than twenty-four hours. "I wasn't sure it was a heart attack, and I didn't want to worry my wife unnecessarily," he said. "I know my blood pressure is high, and I still smoke a little, but I felt fine until this horrible pressure came."

Sam then described the "pressure" as a tightening in his throat and chest, then severe pain that went down his left arm. "When I began to feel nauseated, I knew I should call 911."

Today Sam is a lucky man. Although he did experience a heart attack, because of modern technology he was able to have coronary angioplasty for blocked arteries. But thousands of people each year are not as lucky. Many people like Sam may wonder whether they are having a heart attack, yet ignore the symptoms in the hope that they will go away.

NEVER SECOND-GUESS HEART ATTACK

If you take away anything with you from the reading of this book, it is vital that you learn never to second-guess any symptom that could be related to heart attack. It is far better to hear the doctor say, "There is no problem with your heart" than to wait until there are major problems or until it is too late.

If you experience any of the feelings or signs in chapter 3 that suggest the possibility of coronary heart disease, talk to your doctor immediately. If you happen to have several risk factors for heart disease *and* you suffer chest discomfort, it may be easy for your doctor to tell quickly your risk for heart attack. For example, if you are like Sam, a 60-year-old man who smokes and has hypertension, chest discomfort should be viewed with more suspicion than if you are a 40-year-old man with no other risk factors. The 65-year-old runs a high risk of heart disease, while the 40-year-old's risk may be less than 5 percent.

YOUR DESCRIPTION OF THE WAY YOU FEEL IS IMPORTANT

The way you describe your chest discomfort and the way it behaves will give your doctor clues about whether the cause is heart disease. Certain tests are also available that can usually decide whether the chest discomfort may be from coronary heart disease or whether it may even be safe to ignore it. Everyone does not need every test, but you and your doctor should feel comfortable knowing whether the cause of your chest discomfort is indeed your heart.

"SILENT" ANGINA PECTORIS AND HEART ATTACK

A special problem occurs when coronary heart disease is present but does not cause any chest discomfort at all. These "silent" attacks can be as serious and dangerous as those accompanied by chest discomfort, even though there are no special warning signs. In other words, heart attack, irregular heart beat, and even death may result from these "silent" cases as well. Such attacks can occur during activity and even during rest.

Some researchers have found that most daily angina attacks are actually silent. These often happen when a patient with coronary heart disease is not physically active, but may be under emotional stress. Cigarette smoking has also been found to trigger silent angina attacks in patients who have coronary heart disease. These can be detected when monitoring the heart's response to cigarettes.

Researchers have found that silent angina attacks are more common in the morning hours, which is when blood pressure and heart rate are both higher. It may be that the higher blood pressure and heart rate increase the heart's demand for more blood. When blood supply is insufficient, angina occurs, although it may be "silent."

The exact reasons why some persons do not feel any chest discomfort with angina attacks is not known. The silent attacks are known to occur in diabetes. Since these can be as dangerous as attacks accompanied by chest pain, it becomes even more important that any unusual feelings not be ignored. Proper testing and diagnosis could save your life.

THE ECG (EKG)

If you are experiencing chest discomfort and your doctor suspects heart disease, the electrocardiogram (ECG or EKG) may be one of your first tests. It usually (but not always) registers an abnormal reading during a heart attack. It may be normal even if coronary heart disease is present, especially if done when there is no chest discomfort. If the ECG is abnormal or if your chest discomfort is suspicious for coronary heart disease, further tests may be needed.

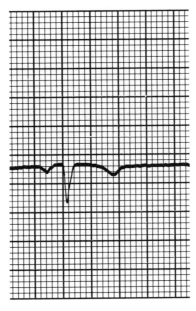

Figure 4.1
A Normal EKG

THE EXERCISE ELECTROCARDIOGRAM OR EXERCISE STRESS TEST

If coronary heart disease is suspected, the next test is often the Exercise Electrocardiogram or Exercise Stress Test. You will be asked to walk, run, or pedal a bicycle while the electrocardiogram is continuously monitored. This goes on until a certain heart rate, depending on age, is reached. A good estimate of your total fitness level will also be available from the exercise.

During the test, your doctor will watch for the response of the heart rate and blood pressure, both of which normally increase during the test. It is also important to monitor whether chest discomfort similar to previous episodes occurs during the exercise. The heart is likewise monitored for irregular heart beats during the exercise test. Although these do commonly occur in healthy persons, the type of irregular beat may be a clue to more serious coronary heart disease.

Certain changes found by your doctor in the electrocardiogram during and after exercise can help predict whether coronary heart disease is present. For example, if the test is normal, the chance of future heart attack is low. The test can help detect coronary heart disease about 75 percent of the time. However, it may erroneously suggest coronary heart disease up to 20 to 25 percent of the time when the heart is normal.

The exercise electrocardiogram can be used in men and women, especially if chest discomfort suggests coronary heart disease. No longer used only with younger patients, it can be helpful in detecting heart disease in persons over sixty-five. It can also help guide the need for further testing, such as cardiac catheterization, and determine later treatment. The exercise electrocardiogram is likewise used for patients who already have coronary heart disease; for example, a low-level exercise test may be used after a heart attack before discharge from the hospital to help plan treatment.

NUCLEAR EXERCISE ELECTROCARDIOGRAM (NUCLEAR EXERCISE TEXT)

In the nuclear exercise electrocardiogram, the exercise test is used just as described above with walking, running, or pedaling a bicycle. The difference is that a special nuclear material such as thallium is injected during the test. Then a series of images of the heart show whether there are any abnormal areas of blood flow in the coronary arteries. The nuclear exercise ECG can show areas of decreased blood flow and sites of possible old heart attacks. Other ways of imaging the heart during this test using computerized tomography can increase the quality of the images and help with accurate diagnosis. This includes SPECT (single photon emission computerized tomography) imaging, which uses computer enhancement to allow more detailed images of the heart.

More accurate than the ordinary ECG, the nuclear exercise ECG increases the ability to detect coronary heart disease to about 85–90 percent. If the nuclear exercise test is normal, your chances of significant heart disease are usually quite low.

IF YOU ARE NOT ABLE TO EXERCISE

If you cannot do enough walking, running or pedaling to perform the exercise test, a medication, dipyridamole, can be injected, which will then be followed by thallium as in the nuclear exercise test described above. This is especially good for patients who suffer from arthritis, back pain, lung disease, or other problems which prevent exercise. The results can be used as in the nuclear exercise test to help decide the best treatment.

Your doctor can tell you which of these tests is the best for your own situation.

CORONARY ANGIOGRAPHY

If the regular exercise or nuclear exercise test is abnormal, then a final test may be needed to decide whether coronary heart disease is actually present. The most accurate test available is coronary angiography, which injects dye directly into the coronary arteries to detect any blockage.

In coronary angiography, small tubes (catheters) are inserted into an artery, usually in the groin, and moved through the arteries into the heart. This is done with the patient awake with very little discomfort. After the contrast dye is injected into the coronary arteries, X-ray images are taken to actually visualize blood flow through the coronary arteries. This can also show how well the heart muscle is pumping blood. Other measurements of the work of the heart can likewise be made during the test.

Coronary angiography testing can help decide the most effective treatment available. For example, results may show that bypass surgery is not needed and that medications would be the best plan of treatment. Or it may give evidence that coronary balloon angioplasty or coronary bypass surgery, as discussed on p. 79, would be advised. Figure 5.1 shows results of coronary angioplasty.

The risks involved in coronary angiography are low. However, because complications may occur, the test is given only to patients whose treatment will be more effective with the new information granted by this treatment. There does exist a small risk that it will worsen the coronary blockage and result in angina pectoris, heart attack, stroke, or bleeding from the groin or other areas. Your doctor can advise you about your own situation.

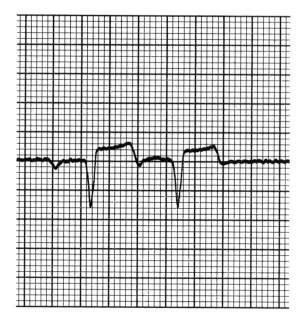

Figure 4.2
Abnormal EKG in a Patient with Heart Attack

TESTS FOR ABNORMAL HEART RHYTHM

In coronary heart disease (as in other types of heart problems), there may be disturbances of the heart rhythm (arrhythmia). In these cases, it may be necessary to evaluate the electrical system that controls the heart's rhythm.

The heart's electrical system usually maintains a smooth and regular rhythm, just as the electrical system of a car engine allows precise distribution of electrical impulses so the car engine runs smoothly.

Electrical problems of the heart can cause the heart rhythm to sputter, beat too fast or irregularly, or in some cases stop completely. These rhythm problems can result in palpitations, which are skipped beats or abnormal sensations of the heartbeat felt in the chest. Not every person feels palpitations. They may be simply annoying or extremely disabling and anxiety-producing.

If the rhythm is irregular, the heart's abnormal pumping action may cause a drop in the blood flow from the heart. This can cause shortness of breath, especially with activity, lightheadedness, dizziness or blackout and loss of consciousness.

Electrocardiogram

The electrocardiogram is usually the first electrical test done to test heart rhythm. Since many abnormal rhythms can be fleeting, it may be difficult to detect the actual disturbance with a standard ECG. Unless the electrical problem is occurring at the time the ECG is taken, it is too difficult to diagnose the problem from the ECG alone.

The Holter Monitor

Another test, called the Holter monitor, allows continuous ECG recording over a 24-hour period. The patient wears a monitor the size of a small purse. This test is very effective in discovering when there are daily episodes of palpitations or other feelings that may be related to abnormal heart beats.

While wearing the monitor, the patient can also make notes in a diary whenever symptoms occur so that later the symptoms can be compared to the heart rhythm at the time of the diary entry. Most monitors have a button on the side, which can be used to mark the recording and precisely identify the time the rhythm happens. By analyzing the results of the 24-hour recording, physicians can direct treatment to correct the abnormal rhythm. However, the abnormal rhythm must occur while the Holter monitor is being worn in order to be detected.

Event Recorder

If the abnormal rhythm does not occur during the wearing of the Holter monitor, another way to reveal any potential problem is with the use of an event recorder. This is a small tape-recording device about the size of a cigarette packet. The device can be worn constantly to record for thirty days or can be carried and simply applied at the time the symptoms develop.

The event recorder can record a short one-to-two-minute ECG which can be transmitted over a telephone line to a central recording station, where the results can be directed to the physician for decisions about treatment. This test allows the physician to see the ECG result within minutes of the development of symptoms. The event recorder is especially helpful when the episodes of abnormal rhythm are infrequent or have been difficult to identify. It is especially helpful for evaluation of patients with blackouts or loss of consciousness.

When Further Testing Is Warranted

If there is still no clear answer to the abnormal rhythm, special testing can be done in a cardiac catheterization laboratory. Electrical wires are inserted through veins into the heart to record electrical impulses. The wires can also be used to create the abnormal rhythm. In this way, the rhythm can be evaluated and treatment planned to eliminate it.

TREATMENT OF ABNORMAL RHYTHM

If the heart rhythm is too slow, some patients benefit from a pacemaker, a small device placed permanently under the skin with a wire connected through a vein to the heart. If the heart rate becomes too slow, the pacemaker automatically begins to stimulate heart rhythm in a way similar to the normal heart pacemaker.

If heart rhythm becomes too fast, it is called tachycardia. Medications are often used to slow and control the heart rate to within the normal range. Because there is a wide range of medications available, the choice of treatment with the least possible side effects is best decided by your doctor.

In some resistant cases, a catheter can be inserted into the heart during electrical testing. The abnormal area producing the rhythm disturbance can be identified and treated, which usually eliminates the abnormal rhythm.

Automatic Implanted Cardioversion Device (AICD)

Some persons with coronary heart disease suffer from sudden episodes of irregular heart rhythm that can cause cardiac arrest and could result in sudden death. These may occur at times without any chest discomfort or heart attack. A good example is the person who collapses while shopping or playing golf. These rhythms are unpredictable and may not be controlled with medications. To treat this problem, a device can be inserted called the Automatic Implanted Cardioversion Device (AICD), which detects abnormal beats and automatically uses an electrical charge to return the heart to normal rhythm.

Using a combination of the above treatments, most patients can experience relief of abnormal heart rhythms.

5

Treating Heart Attack

Winning with heart attack is a reality today. With updated patient information on risk factors as well as the varying diagnostic tests and new modes of treatment available, thousands of heart attack victims each year are surviving and leading normal, active lives.

Mac S. is one such survivor. This 59-year old trial attorney suffered a heart attack more than three years ago. An admitted workaholic, Mac had almost every risk factor on the chart, from high blood pressure to family history to smoking. After he was admitted to the coronary care unit, Mac underwent a series of tests including coronary angiography, which showed four blocked arteries. Mac had coronary artery bypass surgery to correct the blockage. He was discharged after seven days, and after six weeks he returned to work. Mac has now begun to change his risk factors in order to lower his chances of a future heart attack.

This chapter will explain some of the procedures used to treat heart attack. It is our hope that you or a loved one will never have to use these procedures and treatments; but it is important to understand the various treatments should you have a problem. Again, we want to emphasize that if you experience chest discomfort (as described in chapter 3), or if you have unexplained chest discomfort, shortness of breath, or any of the warning signs on p. 54, call your doctor immediately.

CALL 911

When Ted B. suffered a heart attack at age sixty-two, he waited until the last minute to go to the hospital. "I had experienced chest pain before, but the doctor gave me some medicine for that," he told us. "The medicine did not work this time, so I knew I was in trouble."

Instead of calling 911, Ted had his oldest son drive him to a nearby emergency room—through rush hour traffic. "There I sat clutching my chest with perspiration running down my neck, and there my son sat in the midst of a traffic jam. We finally moved on through, but it took a good thirty minutes to go only six miles. They told me several days later that I was lucky I survived, and my doctor emphasized that if this *ever* happened again, that I should immediately call 911."

If you or someone close to you experiences one or more of the symptoms on p. 54, call 911 *immediately* for emergency assistance. Do not take the suspected heart attack victim to the nearest emergency facility in your car. Emergency medical technicians are specially trained and equipped to give initial care to heart attack patients before arrival at the hospital. Their skills can be life-saving, but they need to be granted the opportunity to give service. Remember, the first few hours following a heart attack are extremely important and provide the best opportunity to prevent death. It is critical that there be as little delay as possible between the onset of symptoms and the administration of emergency medical care.

Once emergency medical services arrive on the scene, the heart can be monitored and telephone contact made with the emergency room at the nearest hospital. An intravenous catheter can be inserted in case it is needed for emergency medication. If irregular heart rhythms occur, they can be quickly and effectively treated as the patient is transported for further care.

SUDDEN COLLAPSE

If you are with someone who collapses suddenly, it is important to telephone 911 for emergency help immediately. Six years ago Wilma R., age seventy-four, collapsed while attending a church picnic. Two days earlier Wilma had noticed a sudden shortness of breath and had some tightness in her chest, but ignored these symptoms because she was "too busy." It wasn't until she collapsed that she and her family knew that it was a heart attack. Luckily, Wilma's pastor knew CPR (cardiopulmonary resuscitation) and was able to administer this until emergency personnel arrived.

Wilma's life was saved because of quick action taken by family and friends. It is important to ask for help should someone you know collapse from heart attack. If there is another bystander who knows CPR, he or she should begin immediately while the call for help is being made. Emergency medical personnel will continue CPR if needed, which may include chest compression and electrical shock to restore normal heart rhythm. They will also be sure the patient is breathing properly, assist in keeping the breathing airway open, and give supplemental oxygen. If necessary, a tube will be placed into the airway to allow effective breathing assistance. An intravenous catheter will be inserted for medications. It is crucial to restore oxygen and blood supply in less than four minutes or irreversible brain damage may begin.

After the emergency personnel have established a stable heart rhythm and have restored breathing, the patient will be transported to the nearest hospital emergency room. If necessary, a ventilator (a machine connected to the tube inserted in the throat for breathing) can provide adequate oxygen. The length of hospital stay and the long term outlook will depend on the severity of the heart attack and the length of time the patient went without an adequate blood supply and oxygen to the brain.

CARE IN THE HOSPITAL

If you do suffer a heart attack, it is important to understand what will happen upon arrival in the emergency room. You may expect the following to be done:

- insertion of an intravenous catheter, if not already done

- administration of oxygen by a mask or nasal tube

- medications given under the tongue or by vein

- electrocardiogram (ECG)

- continuous monitoring of the rhythm of the heart for irregular beats

- frequent blood pressure monitoring to be sure treatment can be given if the blood pressure falls or becomes elevated

- questions about your health history and your family's health history

- examination of your heart, other physical examination, and blood tests to help in diagnosis.

After the initial evaluation, if a decision is made to admit you to the hospital, you will be transferred to a bed in the coronary care unit, intensive care unit, or a bed with continuous 24-hour monitoring of the heart available. This precaution is to allow quick treatment in case of irregular heart beat or other complications, especially during the critical first 24-hour time period.

HOW LONG IN HOSPITAL?

A common length of hospitalization for heart attack when there are no complications is four to seven days. After the first day or two you may be transferred from the coronary care or intensive care area to another bed with 24-hour monitoring available. During the hospital stay electrocardiograms will be repeated and other testing may be performed to help decide whether there has been a heart attack, the extent of the heart attack, and what treatment will be needed. You may see a heart specialist (called a cardiologist) in addition to your personal doctor during your hospital stay.

It is important during your time in the hospital that you report any recurrence of chest discomfort, shortness of breath, weakness, dizziness, or other new problems. You will likely begin a cardiac rehabilitation program in which your activities are gradually increased.

Before discharge you may undergo testing such as a low level treadmill exercise or other tests to help decide future risk. This can be done safely under proper supervision, and can help in planning the most effective exercise rehabilitation program when you go home.

At discharge you will be told what your level of activity and exercise should be, how soon you can begin activities such as driving and sexual activity, and when you can return to work. Be sure that you understand any medications your doctor prescribes, any specific diet you should follow, and any other precautions or instructions. Also, be sure you understand when you should next see your doctor for a followup. Your physician may begin to review some risk factors and steps that you can take to prevent heart attack in the future.

A light exercise program begun in the hospital may be continued, often including 5-minute walks performed two to three times daily. This exercise program can be gradually increased under your doctor's direction. You may be advised to enroll in a cardiac rehabilitation program (see p. 39). Some people begin a cardiac rehabilitation program immediately after discharge, while others are instructed to wait for up to six weeks to allow more complete healing of the heart. In such a program you can exercise safely under supervision, including heart monitoring during exercise if needed.

You may notice some weakness, fatigue, or depression once you are at home. These are very common feelings after hospitalization and treatment for coronary heart disease. If these feelings do not quickly fade, be sure your doctor is aware of the problems so that steps can be taken to correct them. While exercise and rehabilitation programs can increase stamina and help to minimize depression, other medical problems and medications needing correction or reevaluation may be contributing factors at times.

Most patients are given the medication nitroglycerin after hospitalization to be used in the event of further chest discomfort. Nitroglycerin is a tablet that helps to provide improved blood supply to the heart. If you experience chest discomfort, you should sit down and place one nitroglycerin tablet under your tongue (or use the nitroglycerin spray). If relief does not occur within five minutes, place another nitroglycerin under your tongue. If pain persists after an additional five minutes, place another nitroglycerin tablet under your tongue, and call your doctor immediately or go to the nearest emergency room.

During your doctor's visits after hospital treatment, your blood pressure and pulse will be closely monitored. Your doctor will listen to your heart and lungs to ensure that the medications you are taking are correct and necessary at the time. There will be more discussion of control of risk factors and any changes necessary to reduce your risk of future heart attack (see chapter 6).

Remember to bring a list of your medications or the medication bottles themselves to your regular visits with your doctor. This will help to maintain accurate communication about proper medication. If a medication is added during your visit, be sure you receive the appropriate prescription.

The frequency of return visits to your doctor will vary according to your condition and rate of improvement. Some patients may find it necessary to see their doctor only once a year.

PROLONGED CHEST DISCOMFORT
AND UNSTABLE ANGINA PECTORIS

If you experience chest discomfort that lasts for more than twenty minutes, you should strongly consider medical evaluation at the nearest medical facility. This prolonged chest discomfort may be the only warning sign you have of a serious heart problem. If you have already had a heart attack or coronary heart disease, then it may be necessary for you to be monitored for twenty-four hours in a hospital to make sure heart attack or other damage does not occur.

If you have angina pectoris (described on p. 54), and you begin to experience more frequent discomfort *or* the pain comes on with much less activity than usual, *or* if the pain occurs while you are at rest, then you may have unstable angina. In unstable angina pectoris you need immediate medical evaluation and hospital observation to be sure heart attack or other problems such as irregular rhythm are detected and treated properly.

MEDICATIONS FOR TREATMENT

A large number of medications are available to treat coronary heart disease. Some of those most commonly used are listed on pp. 93–97. These medications may also be given intravenously during hospital treatment.

Nitrates (Nitroglycerin and Others)

Nitrates help decrease the heart's need for oxygen and improve the supply of oxygen to the heart muscle. They can be given under the tongue, by skin patch, by tablet, or intravenously.

Beta Blockers

Beta blockers help reduce the heart's need for oxygen and commonly lower the heart rate.

Calcium Antagonists

Calcium antagonists can both reduce the heart's need for oxygen and increase the supply of oxygen to the heart from the arteries.

Aspirin

Aspirin has been used in low doses to reduce the risk of sudden blockage of coronary arteries, which can result in the worsening of heart attack or angina pectoris. It is also used in longer term prevention of heart attack, as discussed on p. 112.

Clot-Dissolving Medications

Medications are used to dissolve clots in the coronary arteries, resulting from heart attack and unstable angina pectoris. These medications attempt to dissolve the clot (thrombosis) in the coronary artery, commonly found in heart attack. The goals of this treatment are to decrease the size or severity of the heart attack and to lower the chance of permanent heart damage and death.

These medications are given intravenously. The most common are tissue plasminiogen activator (TPA) and streptokinase. Side effects are possible, including the risk of bleeding, so patients are monitored very closely during treatment.

OTHER TREATMENT FOR CORONARY HEART DISEASE

Percutaneous Transluminal Coronary Angioplasty (PTCA)

Depending on the type of blockage found on coronary angiography, this procedure can be used in stable angina pectoris, unstable angina pectoris, or acute myocardial infarction. In PTCA a catheter, after insertion in the artery in the groin, is placed into the coronary artery as in coronary angiography (discussed on p. 67). A wire is placed in the blocked artery and a balloon catheter is inflated at the site of the blockage to expand the arterial opening.

The expansion of the balloon crushes the thickened material that extends into the artery (see figure 5.1). There is also some mild injury to the wall of the coronary artery. Researchers have found healing of the injury to the wall of the artery after about one month.

About 90 percent of patients have good results from PTCA with blockage of the artery reduced by 50 percent or more. PTCA has been used with increasing success; in 1992, more than 300,000 people underwent PTCA.

Complications are uncommon but heart attack or the need to proceed with emergency coronary bypass surgery can occur in about 5 percent or less of patients who have PTCA. In about eight out of every one hundred patients who undergo PTCA, the artery may close again within twenty-four hours. Bleeding from the site of insertion of the catheter and other problems in the arteries of the extremities occur in a few cases. Recurrence of the blockage may happen in about 30 percent of cases after three to six months.

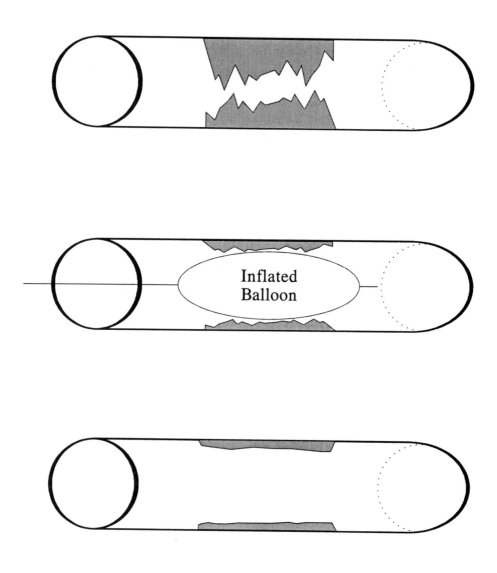

Figure 5.1
How PTCA expands the blocked artery

Every person is different. Your doctor can give you specific advice regarding your own case.

Coronary Artery Bypass Surgery

Some patients have blockages in coronary arteries which are too extensive or otherwise not suitable for PTCA. Depending on the type of coronary artery blockage, surgery may be recommended.

Coronary bypass surgery is reserved for those patients whose symptoms cannot be controlled with medication and who would not benefit from angioplasty (PTCA). The surgery is performed when there is a blockage in one or more coronary arteries, too extensive for angioplasty but with an open artery after the blockage. The mortality rate is low, usually about 1 percent, but can be higher in emergency surgery, in unstable angina pectoris, and in older patients. The hospital stay is often about seven days.

Coronary bypass surgery is successful in over 80 percent of patients who have unstable angina pectoris who are not controlled by medical treatment. In addition, if successful, the surgery may help prevent heart attack in the future. Severe blockage of coronary arteries alone does not mean bypass surgery will be helpful. The arteries must also be able to carry the new blood supply to the heart muscle after the bypass is completed.

Some of the most common complications after bypass surgery include heart attack, blockage of the newly grafted blood vessel, and worsening of the atherosclerosis in the arteries. Up to half of patients may develop blockages in other parts of the arteries after five years.

A portion of a vein from a leg is used to reroute the flow of blood. The vein is inserted (grafted) from the aorta past the area of blockage into the coronary artery (see figure 5.2). Or, an artery from the chest, the internal mammary artery, is used to supply blood past the blockage in the artery. Studies now show that results can be good even in many patients age seventy and older. Other factors are also important, such as how well the heart pumps and whether other serious medical problems are present.

Coronary artery bypass surgery has been demonstrated to give relief in angina pectoris. Some studies have shown improvement in coronary blockage and less risk of death from heart attack among patients who have undergone this treatment. A combination of treatments is best.

Each person is different. Your doctor will guide you so that you receive the most effective combination of medical treatment and surgery available. Then begin to prevent future heart disease as outlined in chapter 6.

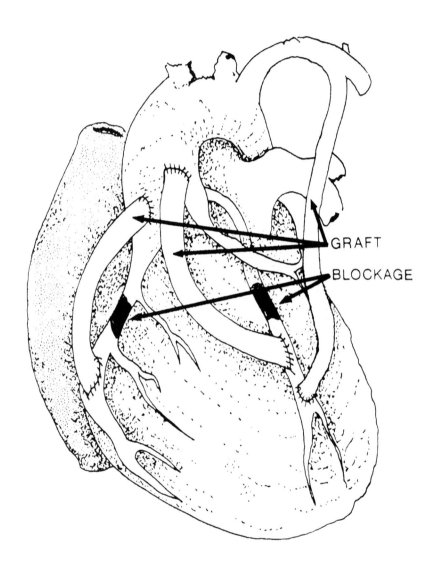

Figure 5.2
Parts of a vein from a leg or an artery can be used to
reroute blood past a blockage in a coronary artery.

6

A Prevention Plan for Heart Attack

Thirty years ago, heart attack may have been an expected reality for many older adults. But with new medical technology for treatment and a greater understanding of risk factors that contribute to cardiovascular disease, heart attack prevention can occur in your lifetime. And the earlier you begin to manage your lifestyle to prevent heart attack, the more effective the results will be. Action taken early in life may produce better results than action taken later, when cardiovascular disease is already present.

ASSESS YOUR RISK FACTORS

After carefully reading chapter 2, fill in the blanks on p. 51 to determine your personal set of risk factors for heart attack. This chapter will teach you ways to begin necessary steps to control these risk factors or eliminate them altogether. After completing this chapter, use the form on p. 52 to set personal goals as you begin a plan to lessen your chances of heart attack. Remember: the more risk factors you have, the greater the risk for cardiovascular disease and the more reason to get started immediately to *halt heart attack*.

Controlling risk factors to *prevent* coronary heart disease is the best approach today. But even if you have already suffered angina pectoris or heart attack, there is now good evidence that you can take steps to stop or *reverse* the process in the coronary arteries. For example, studies show that if you reduce your cholesterol levels, stop smoking, and add cardiac exercise programs, you can lower your chances of having a serious or possibly fatal heart attack.

There is so much to gain by taking charge of your health and well-being. The prevention techniques we address in this chapter do not require a drastic lifestyle change; in fact, most people are able to incorporate healthy, low-fat eating along with an exercise program into their daily schedules. Other lifestyle changes such as cutting back on salt in your diet, limiting alcohol, adding heart-healthy foods, and taking medication, if needed, to control hypertension and cholesterol are not difficult. Indeed, most people who begin making changes to protect their heart health tell of feeling better than ever. They are more physically active, have more energy, lose excess weight, and feel younger. You can improve the limitations and possible fatal outcome of coronary heart disease once you know the specific steps to take.

CONTROL HYPERTENSION

If you have hypertension, you are not alone: it affects 50 to 60 million Americans. By controlling your hypertension you can reduce the suffering and disability from other diseases and help lower the nation's health care costs. It can be done with a minimum of trouble and expense, and many times even without medication.

You may ask: When is blood pressure too high and when should it be treated? Some studies show that as blood pressure increases above 120/80, there is a corresponding risk of cardiovascular disease.

If your blood pressure is less than 130 systolic and less than 85 diastolic, it is in the normal range. If your blood pressure is 130–139 systolic or 85–89 diastolic, then it is high normal and you should recheck your pressure at least every few months to be sure it does not grow higher.

The primary goal in treating hypertension is to bring the readings to normal levels or as close to normal as possible, and to do so with the fewest possible side effects. Many find that their blood pressure will fall within to the normal range with easy steps for treatment without medication.

When medications are needed, goals are to use the least expensive medication possible that gives the desired results and allows the fewest possible doses each day. Remember that blood pressure can be controlled with medication safely and effectively without significant side effects in most cases!

Borderline Systolic Hypertension

Systolic blood pressure between 140 and 160 but normal diastolic blood pressure has been called *borderline systolic hypertension*. Information now shows that these readings commonly increase to definite hypertension. Readings at this level should be rechecked every one to two weeks. After you talk with your doctor, you may decide to begin some of ways of lowering blood pressure and removing this risk factor without medication.

Systolic Hypertension

For years it was assumed that systolic blood pressure was not important for future risk, being less important than the diastolic reading. Researchers have now shown that systolic hypertension is at least as important as diastolic in determining future risk.

When systolic blood pressure levels are above normal, add treatment without medication to lower the systolic blood pressure to normal levels. In many cases these steps will be enough. If blood pressure does not fall below 140, medication may also be needed. Talk to your doctor.

Diastolic Hypertension

If your diastolic blood pressure remains normal (below 85) then check it yearly. If it reads 85 to 89 after several readings, then check the reading at least every one to two months to be sure it doesn't increase. Check your risk factors and review your steps to lower blood pressure without medications as discussed below.

Treatment without medication lowers the diastolic blood pressure in many cases. But if the diastolic pressure does not return to less than 90, then medication may also be needed.

TREATMENT OF HYPERTENSION WITHOUT MEDICATION

Following are some important lifestyle changes that can be made to reduce hypertension without medication. Ask your doctor if these would be useful for you.

1. Lower Your Salt Intake to Lower Blood Pressure

Some people with hypertension find that lowering their salt and sodium intake can lower their blood pressure. This is especially true for those who are used to excess salt in their diet and those who happen to be sensitive to the effects of salt on blood pressure. It is not known why some are more sensitive to this intake than others. Lowering the amount of salt often works to allow you to reduce medication or even avoid it altogether.

It isn't very hard to reduce excess salt intake in the diet and there are no serious side effects. This can be an important first step in treating hypertension.

Salt in the diet should be restricted to 2 grams of sodium per day; this is called a "no-added salt diet." One teaspoon of salt contains about 2 grams of sodium.

Do Not Add Salt to Foods

First, simply *stop adding salt* to your food at the table. The food may still be cooked with a normal amount of salt, but don't cheat by increasing the salt in cooking. Your taste will definitely change so that you actually enjoy less salt. Soon the recipes you used to enjoy will taste too salty. This is a painless way to lower salt intake for many of us. The more trouble you have breaking this habit, the more excess salt you may be taking in your diet—and the greater your need to accomplish this change.

Avoid Foods Known to Have Excess Salt

Next, *avoid foods known to contain excess salt.* Many foods may have much more sodium than you would expect, even though they may not taste very salty. For example, did you know that many canned soups contain more sodium than is needed for an entire day? Many snack foods, prepared foods, and fast foods also have large amounts of salt. Now this doesn't mean you must give them up forever. Just begin to avoid them when you have a choice.

Check the list in table 6.1. By restricting your intake of high-sodium prepared and fast foods, you will soon find that your taste will change and that some old favorites will soon taste more salty, less appealing, and easier to set aside.

Table 6.1
Foods High in Sodium

Food	Amount	Milligrams*
American cheese	1 slice	260
Bacon	2 slices	600
Bacon bits	2 tbsp.	430
Beef bouillon	1 cube	1150
Biscuit with sausage	125 g	1100
Cheeseburger, fast food	¼ lb.	1200
Chicken noodle soup	1 cup	1100
Chicken sandwich, fast food	1	750
Chile con carne	8 oz.	1100
Cottage cheese	1 cup	625
Danish roll, cheese	1 medium	420
Fish sandwich, fast food	1 reg.	750
Garlic salt	1 tsp.	1850
Ham	3 oz.	1000
Hot cakes (3) with butter	180 g	650
Luncheon meat	1 slice	575
Macaroni and cheese	1 cup	700
Meat tenderizer	1 tsp.	1750
Olives, green	3	720
Onion salt	1 tsp.	1620
Oyster stew	1 cup	940
Peas, green canned	1 cup	493
Pizza, cheese	⅛ of 14″	525
Potato, instant	1 cup	475
Salt	¼ tsp.	500
Sauerkraut	⅔ cup	740
Soy sauce	1 tbsp.	1030
Tuna, canned	3 oz.	700
Vegetable juice	11.5 oz. can	980

---

*One thousand milligrams is equivalent to one gram. The American Heart Association recommends no more than 1000 to 3000 milligrams (mg) sodium per day.

There are many herbs and spices that can be used effectively to increase taste and decrease sodium. If you have questions about or have trouble breaking the salt habit, talk to your doctor, who can help you contact a dietician or nutritionist (see also chapter 7).

2. Control Your Weight to Lower Blood Pressure

Being overweight increases your chance of hypertension. A great way to help control your blood pressure is to begin a weight loss program. Even losing five to ten pounds may have a significant effect in lowering your blood pressure. The best combination for weight loss is to lower your calorie intake in a comfortable way so that you are not hungry, as discussed in chapter 7, and gradually increase exercise. It isn't as hard as it seems if you do it sensibly and slowly. But it is always a good idea to discuss weight loss with your doctor before you begin.

Control Calorie Intake

To lose weight, you must take in fewer calories than you consume in your daily activity. There is no way to avoid this: You must either lower your calorie intake or burn more calories to allow weight loss. Diets that promise weight loss without calorie reduction are simply fooling you.

Figure 6.1
Balanced Weight Loss

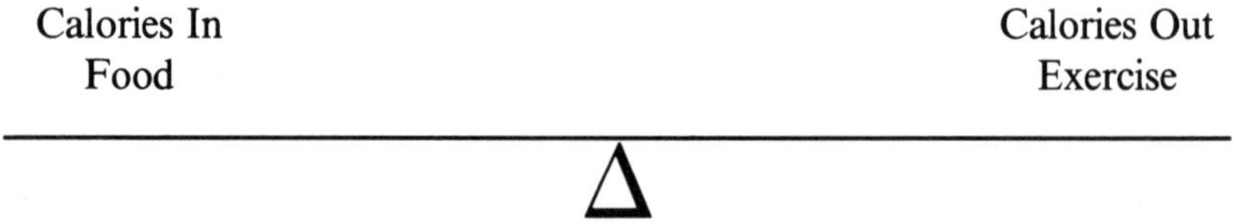

Calories In		Calories Out
Food		Exercise

$$\Delta$$

Increase Calories Used

You can burn more calories with exercise, and so lose weight. An easy way to begin is with a walking program. Simply walk a short distance daily, gradually increasing the distance. If you lose one-half to one pound each week, you're doing enough walking. If you don't lose that much, then increase the distance or time you walk until you maintain the right balance between exercise and calories to lose one-half to one pound each week. If you already have heart disease, be especially sure your doctor approves of the walking program before you start.

If You Can't Lose Weight

If you don't seem able to lose weight, then it is important to find out why. If there are no other medical problems present, you may need help in lowering your calorie intake. Suppressing your appetite with medication or using a very low calorie diet (400–600 calories per day) may be short-term but less desirable ways to begin weight loss in a few selected cases.

Weight loss is a long-term plan. Don't give up if you can't see results immediately. It is simply a matter of finding which weight loss program will work for you. The best weight loss program we have seen is described in chapter 7: our patients find it to be an easy, painless, and effective way to lose weight gradually and permanently.

3. Begin a Regular Exercise Program to Lower Blood Pressure

Blood pressure can also be lowered with a regular exercise program. Many types of exercise, such as walking or bicycling, fit well into a plan of gradual weight loss. After checking first with your doctor, choose an exercise that is convenient and that you enjoy (or at least don't mind) doing. If you hate an exercise or find it inconvenient, you probably won't continue it very long.

If your schedule limits your time for exercise, you may need to consider an exercise program you can do at home, such as with a treadmill or an exercise bicycle. This would allow you to exercise anytime, day or night, regardless of the weather. Other possibilities include swimming, jogging, or jumping rope. These provide excellent exercise in a short time.

Be Sure to Start Slowly

Begin your exercise program with one to two minutes per session once each day so that you are not tired afterward. Then gradually increase up to fifteen to twenty minutes a day or more, five days a week.

If you have heart disease, it may be a good idea to join a cardiac rehabilitation program when you start your exercise. This allows you to exercise under supervision, and if needed, your heart can be monitored during exercise.

4. Manage Stress to Lower Blood Pressure

Emotional stress and anxiety from job, family, and other problems can raise blood pressure. If stress is contributing to your hypertension, some easy steps for stress management might lower it.

One way is a *regular exercise program.* Exercise can lower stress, which may itself improve blood pressure.

Some other excellent ways to improve your control of stress include *relaxation response* techniques discussed on pp. 146–49. These can be learned and have been shown to relax muscles, lower blood pressure, and lower heart rate.

Read about the feelings of stress described on pp. 42–44. If you realize stress is a factor in your life that needs to be controlled more effectively, take some tips from chapter 8. These tips help reduce your tension—and may lower your blood pressure as well!

5. Lower Excess Alcohol Intake to Lower Blood Pressure

Although low to moderate amounts of alcohol, especially wine, may actually reduce the risk of heart attack, when alcohol intake increases above the equivalent of about three drinks per day (see pp. 33–34), the chance of hypertension increases. If you find you can't limit your intake to a healthy amount, it would be better to stop alcohol altogether. Check with your doctor to see whether any specific limits on alcohol are needed in your particular situation.

6. Have an Adequate Intake of Potassium and Calcium to Lower Blood Pressure

When your intake of the mineral potassium is low, bringing the level up to normal can help reduce blood pressure. This step to reduce hypertension is probably not as important as other steps such as lowering the amount of sodium in your diet. Taking extra potassium supplements is not usually necessary unless your diet is low in potassium or you are on a medication that causes low potassium. Many foods such as cantaloupe, orange juice, bananas, potatoes, and others listed in table 6.2 contain natural potassium. Don't increase your potassium unless you check with your doctor to make sure it is safe for you. Higher than normal levels of potassium in the blood can cause abnormal heart rhythm.

Table 6.2
Foods High in Potassium

Apricots (fresh)	Milk (whole)
Apricots (dried)	Orange juice
Avocados	Peaches
Bananas	Potatoes
Buttermilk	Raisins
Cantaloupe	Salmon (fresh cooked)
Chicken	Sardines
Cod	Sweet potatoes
Flounder	Tomatoes (raw)
Great Northern beans (cooked)	Turkey
Milk (skim)	

Increases in calcium intake in some persons may lower their blood pressure (see table 6.3). It is a good idea to be sure you have the recommended daily allowance for calcium: The recommended daily allowance for calcium for adult men and women is 1000 mg per day; for women after menopause, 1500 mg per day. However, higher than normal calcium levels in the blood can cause serious medical problems, so don't increase your calcium intake to levels higher than recommended without your doctor's advice.

Table 6.3
Foods High in Calcium

Food	Amount	Milligrams
Beans:		
Baked	1 cup	150
Black	1 cup	270
Beets (steamed)	1 cup	145
Broccoli (steamed)	1 cup	135
Chard (steamed, leaves)	1 cup	130
Cheese:		
American cheese spread	1 oz.	175
Cheddar	1 oz.	210
Cottage cheese	2%	150
Parmesan	1 tbsp.	65

Table 6.3
Foods High in Calcium (cont'd.)

Sliced (American)	1 oz.	150–280
Swiss	1 oz.	270–300
Collards (steamed)	1 cup	35
Dandelion greens (steamed)	1 cup	300
Garbanzo beans (canned)	1 cup	150
Ice cream (most flavors)	1 cup	150
Kale (steamed)	1 cup	205
Mustard greens (steamed)	1 cup	200
Okra (steamed)	1 cup	150
Salmon (canned)	3 oz.	160–250
Sardines (canned with bones)	8 med.	350–450
Soybeans	1 cup	130
Spinach (steamed)	1 cup	170
Turnip greens (steamed)	1 cup	270
Watercress (raw, finely chopped)	1 cup	190
Yogurt		
nonfat	8 oz.	450
1.5% fat	8 oz.	350

TREATMENT OF HYPERTENSION WITH MEDICATION

If treatment without medication does not lower your blood pressure to the normal range in a few months, there are many medications available that can help you control it without side effects. One point is clear: control hypertension and you can lower your risk of coronary heart disease.

When should hypertension be treated with medications? Each case is different; but before seeking medication, try all the steps outlined for *treatment without medication,* including lowering your salt intake, controlling your weight, maintaining a regular exercise program, decreasing alcohol intake, and managing stress.

1. If your diastolic blood pressure is still 85–89, then check the pressure every one to two months to make sure it doesn't increase further. If your diastolic blood pressure is still 90 or higher after a few months, then *treating with medications* to lower the blood pressure to normal levels may be needed. Your doctor can advise you about medications,

but be sure to continue the steps for treatment without medication. Treatment is especially needed if other risk factors for coronary heart disease are present.

2. If your diastolic blood pressure remains 95 or greater, medications to control blood pressure are needed. Be sure to continue the regime of treatment without medications as well.

3. If your systolic blood pressure is between 140 and 159, continue treatment without medications. However, many physicians would consider adding medication to lower your blood pressure to 140 or less, especially if you have other risk factors or if you already have heart disease.

4. If your systolic blood pressure is 160 or above, then in addition to the methods for treatment without medication, you should consider adding medication to your lower blood pressure. The goal is to reduce blood pressure to normal levels (below 140) or as close as possible without side effects.

5. If your diastolic blood pressure is 110 or greater, *see your physician immediately for treatment.*

Medications Available for Treatment of Hypertension

A large number of medications are available to treat hypertension. For many years, diuretics which cause high urine discharge were the drugs of choice to treat hypertension. These are often effective, may be taken in one dose daily, and are usually safe. They are among the lowest priced of the available medications.

One concern is that diuretics' side effects may include decreased potassium, which can contribute to irregular heart rhythms. There is also concern that even if diuretic treatment lowers blood pressure, it may offer less protective effect for coronary heart disease. This is because in large studies there was less reduction in coronary heart disease than expected when diuretics were used for treatment of hypertension.

Over the past twenty years many other medications have become available to treat hypertension. The large number of choices offers almost everyone the possibility of maintaining good blood pressure control without side effects. Many of these medications may be taken only once each day, which makes correct dosage easier to remember. However, the newer medications may be more expensive.

If your blood pressure is not controlled within one to three months after starting on the medication, your doctor may choose to *increase the dose* of the same medication, *replace* the medication, or *add* a second medication. Treatment is individualized to offer the best possible control of blood pressure with the fewest side effects. This may require some patience in order to find the proper combination of medication for your own situation. Twenty to 40 percent of patients may need to stop or change medications because of side effects or for better control of blood pressure. Some of the most common medications used to control hypertension are listed on pp. 93ff.

Medications being taken for other reasons, such as anti-inflammatory drugs for arthritis, may alter the effect of some blood pressure medications or may increase the chance of side effects. Check with your doctor.

Side Effects of Medications

Practically every medicine has potential side effects. When you take any medication, it should be for a specific purpose—and side effects are always possible. If the benefits outweigh the possible side effects, then the medication may be taken. As discussed in chapter 2, the dangers of uncontrolled hypertension and heart disease outweigh the risks of medications for most people.

Some of the most common side effects of medications used in the control of blood pressure are listed with the medications given below. Twenty to 40 percent of patients may need to stop or change medications because of side effects or for better control of blood pressure.

While a few of the most common side effects are noted in this volume, a more complete list of possible side effects can be found in the package insert provided with each medication. Remember that everyone is different and may react differently to each medication. Check with your doctor for any specific side effects and their treatment.

Don't hesitate to report side effects to your doctor. While most people do not suffer from side effects, it is important to watch for any unexplained problems. Many problems may not even be related to the medication, but your doctor would still want to know about any difficulties you are experiencing with the medication. If a problem is in fact caused by your medication, it may be resolved by changing the dosage or using a different medication.

Weakness and sexual problems, especially in men, can occur with any of the medications. There are many other causes of these symptoms, however, and there may be other problems present which need to be discovered and corrected.

If you have *any* questions or concerns about your medications or other steps you are taking to control your hypertension, then get more information.

When Blood Pressure Becomes Normalized

Once normalized, your blood pressure should be measured regularly to make sure good control is maintained. Measurements might be weekly at first, then less often when pressure remains normal. It may be a good idea to measure your blood pressure at home in order to get an idea of how it varies during the day.

Your doctor can tell you how often you need to be seen to ensure side effects are not a problem. This could be as little as once each year. Blood tests may be needed occasionally when taking some medications to check for side effects.

Be prepared to continue medications for hypertension over a long period of time. After one year of normal blood pressure it may be possible to lower or stop medication, but only under your doctor's supervision. Don't stop your medication (even though you feel "just fine") without first talking with your doctor.

It is important that you *never* run out of medicine. Keep a supply at home, and try to refill the prescription before it runs out. Without medication, your blood pressure may rise suddenly and cause serious problems, such as stroke or heart attack. None of these medications should be used during pregnancy without your doctors' advice.

SOME OF THE MOST COMMON MEDICATIONS FOR HYPERTENSION

Diuretics

Brand Name	Generic Name
Dyrenium, Dyazide, Maxide	Triamterene/Hydrochlorthiazide
Hydrodiuril	Hydrochlorthiazide
Lasix	Furosemide
Bumex	Bumetanide
Lozol	Indapamide
Diuril	Chlorthiazide
Hygroton	Chlorthalidone

Diuretics (cont'd.)

Brand Name	*Generic Name*
Moduretic	Amiloride
Zaroxolyn	Metolazone
Euduron	Methyclothiazide
Salutensin	Hydroflumethazide
Naturetin	Bendroflumethiazide
Aldactone	Spironolactone
Naqua	Trichlormethiazide
Edecrin	Ethacrynic Acid

Note: Some diuretics can cause low potassium, low sodium, higher glucose, and higher cholesterol and triglycerides. Some that are intended to prevent low potassium (the first line on the list above) may also cause potassium to increase to high levels. Your doctor can tell you how often you should be checked for potassium level and side effects.

Beta Blockers

Brand Name	*Generic Name*
Tenormin	Atenolol
Lopressor	Metoprolol
Corgard	Nadolol
Inderal	Propranolol
Blocadren	Timolol

Beta Blockers with Sympathomimetic Activity

Brand Name	*Generic Name*
Sectral	Acebotolol
Cartrol	Carteolol
Levatol	Penbutolol
Viskin	Pindolol

Note: Beta blockers lower blood pressure and heart rate by interfering with the effects of adrenalin. They can cause fatigue, and can aggravate asthma or congestive heart failure. They also can cause higher triglycerides and lower HDL cholesterol. They must be used with caution in persons with heart and lung disease, diabetes mellitus, and diseases of the arteries in the feet and legs. They should not be stopped suddenly in persons with coronary heart disease, but gradually lowered in dose before stopping, to avoid aggravation of heart problems. Beta blockers with sympathomimetic activity reduce blood pressure by effect on the heart, with less slowing of the heart rate.

Alpha-Beta Blocker

Brand Name	*Generic Name*
Normodyne, Trandate	Labetalol

Note: Alpha-beta blockers reduce blood pressure by their effect on the heart and blood vessels. They should be used with caution in persons with heart disease, asthma or other lung disease, diabetes mellitus, or diseases of the arteries in the feet and legs.

Alpha 1 Receptor Blockers

Brand Name	*Generic Name*
Cardura	Doxazosin
Minipres	Prazosin
Hytrin	Terazosin

Note: Alpha 1 receptor blockers lower blood pressure by their effect on blood vessels. They can cause dizziness from a drop in blood pressure on standing, weakness, palpitations, and headache. They are used with caution in older patients because of the possible drop in blood pressure on standing.

ACE Inhibitors

Brand Name	*Generic Name*
Vasotec	Enalapril
Prinivil, Zestril	Lisinopril
Lotensin	Benazepril
Capoten	Captopril
Monopril	Fosinopril

ACE Inhibitors (cont'd.)

Brand Name	*Generic Name*
Accupril	Quinapril
Altace	Ramipril

Note: ACE inhibitors lower blood pressure by interfering with the action of angiotensin converting enzyme, which is normally present in the body but can contribute to hypertension. These medications can cause cough, rash, high potassium levels, or other problems. They should not be used during pregnancy without your doctor's advice.

Calcium Antagonists

Brand Name	*Generic Name*
Cardizem, Dilacor	Diltiazem
Calan, Isoptin, Verelan	Verapimil
Norvasc	Amlodipine
Plendil	Felodipine
DynaCirc	Isradipine
Cardene	Nicardipine
Procardia, Adalat	Nifedipine

Note: Calcium antagonists decrease the amount of calcium flowing into muscle cells of the arteries, keeping them more relaxed. They can cause headache, dizziness, edema (a buildup of fluid in the body tissues), rapid heart rate, or constipation. They are used with caution in patients with heart disease.

Centrally Acting Medications

Brand Name	*Generic Name*
Catapres	Clonidine
Wytensin	Guanabenz
Tenex	Guanfacine
Aldomet	Methlydopa

Note: Centrally acting agents are thought to work by their action on chemicals in the brain which in turn lower blood pressure. They can cause drowsiness, mouth dryness, fatigue, and dizziness. Blood tests may be needed at intervals to check for side effects. Suddenly stopping the medication can result in rebound elevation of blood pressure.

Peripheral Acting Agents

Brand Name	Generic Name
Hylorel	Guanadrel
Esimil	Guanethidine
Generic Brand	Reserpine

Note: Peripheral acting agents lower blood pressure by interfering with chemicals that stimulate blood vessels. They can cause diarrhea, dizziness on standing, fatigue, nasal congestion, and depression. They should be avoided in persons with depression or active peptic ulcer.

Direct Vasodilators

Brand Name	Generic Name
Apresoline	Hydralazine
Loniten	Minoxidil

Note: Direct vasodilators lower blood pressure by expanding and relaxing blood vessels. They can cause headache, rapid heart rate, and fluid retention, and must be used with caution in persons with heart disease. Minoxidil can also cause increase in hair on the face and other areas.

CONTROL ABNORMAL CHOLESTEROL AND TRIGLYCERIDES

As discussed in chapter 2, abnormal blood cholesterol is one of the most important risk factors for heart attack. The risk of heart disease gradually increases along with the cholesterol. The levels of LDL cholesterol, HDL cholesterol and triglycerides are the most important for determining heart risk. Check the guides for treatment recommendations from the National Cholesterol Education Project.

Table 6.4
Treatment Recommendations for Controlling Cholesterol

If Your Number Is:

LDL cholesterol over 100 and you have coronary heart disease	Begin diet
LDL cholesterol over 130 and two or more risk factors	Begin diet
LDL cholesterol over 160	Begin diet

If you have coronary heart disease and your numbers are still above these levels after six to twelve weeks of the Step II diet (see p. 99), then consider adding medication. If you do not have coronary heart disease and your numbers are still abnormal after six months of Step I or Step II diet, then consider adding medication.

After Heart Attack, Controlling Cholesterol May Be Even More Important

Studies show that *lowering LDL cholesterol* and *raising HDL cholesterol* can help to decrease heart attacks. After the first heart attack, it may be even more helpful to lower cholesterol, since it has been shown that it is possible in many cases to stop or reverse the blockage of the coronary arteries.

Use an Easy Diet to Control Cholesterol and Triglycerides

An estimated 52 million adults in America need to follow a diet to help control their cholesterol. Many respond to a diet as described in chapter 7, which painlessly lowers saturated fat (mainly animal and dairy fats), raises certain polyunsaturated fats (some vegetable oils) and adds monounsaturated fats (like olive oil).

The proper diet involves knowing which foods to choose and which to avoid. It can be followed by using a polyunsaturated margarine, olive oil, low fat milk (skim or 1 or 2 percent), eating more fish and poultry; sticking to lean meat; and eating more fresh fruits, vegetables, and fiber (see table 6.5).

If it's too much for you to change all parts of your diet at once, choose one or two areas that seem easiest and begin slowly. For example, start by using a polyunsaturated margarine in place of butter, or more olive oil in cooking. These are painless alternatives that can make a real difference.

Table 6.5
Some Easy Diet Steps in Controlling Cholesterol

- use polyunsaturated margarine such as safflower or corn oil
- use olive oil in cooking
- use low fat milk (skim, 1%, 2%)
- eat more fish and poultry
- use only lean and fat trimmed meat
- eat more fresh fruits and vegetables
- add more fiber to your diet

Step I and Step II Diets Can
Control Cholesterol and Lower Triglycerides

A Step I diet recommended by the National Cholesterol Education Program and American Heart Association to lower cholesterol and triglycerides includes:

- 30 percent of calories from fat
- less than 10 percent of calories from saturated fats
- up to 10 percent of calories from polyunsaturated fats
- up to 15 percent of calories from monosaturated fats
- and less than 300 mg cholesterol per day.

A Step II diet can be used if the Step I diet does not control the abnormal cholesterol and triglycerides. It provides:

- less than 7 percent of calories from saturated fats
- and less than 200 mg cholesterol.

These diets can lower total cholesterol, LDL cholesterol and triglycerides and help in weight control. If they are not effective or you simply can't follow them closely enough to bring the levels to the desired range, then medication may have to be considered.

These diets also lower cholesterol in most cases over a period of three to six months. For those who don't want to give up meat, studies show that meat can be part of a diet to control cholesterol if it is lean and the outer fat or skin is carefully trimmed.

Don't Feel Guilty

Many people suffer guilt if their cholesterol level does not drop low enough with diet. They feel that their doctors might believe they aren't cooperating unless their cholesterol improves. Diet does not control cholesterol in all cases! In fact, it is estimated that at least 13 million people need medication as well. If you follow the diet as closely as you possibly can, then don't feel guilty if your cholesterol level does not become normal. Your best effort at diet is good enough.

Increase Omega-3 and Omega-6 Fats

Increasing your intake of omega-3 fats can lower the LDL cholesterol if it is high, and help raise HDL cholesterol. Omega-3 fats are found in certain fish or in supplements called EPA (elcosapentaenoic acid), or fish oil capsules found in your pharmacy or health food store. See the list of foods containing omega-3 fats on p. 125.

Increasing your intake of omega-6 fats lowers LDL cholesterol, but in higher amounts can also lower HDL cholesterol, which would not be desirable because of its heart protective effect. These fats are found in certain vegetable oils such as safflower oil.

Use Monounsaturated Fats

Using monounsaturated fats in the diet (easily done by using olive oil), especially when these replace saturated fats, can lower cholesterol overall by lowering LDL cholesterol. Monounsaturated fats do not lower HDL cholesterol, which is good for the heart.

Add Antioxidants

Adding antioxidants to your diet can help protect against the effect of oxidants, which are normally produced by chemical reactions in the body. Oxidants can damage cells and are thought to damage LDL cholesterol, thus making it more harmful in the arteries in atherosclerosis. Fruits and vegetables, vitamin E, beta carotene (found in carrots, sweet potatoes, and cantaloupe), and vitamin C are good sources of anti-oxidants.

Garlic May Help

Some other specific diet items may help lower cholesterol. For example, there is evidence that garlic added to the diet may help. Some results show at least a 9 percent reduction in cholesterol using the equivalent of one-half to one clove of garlic per day. This can also be taken in the form of pills.

Does Fiber Help the Heart?

There is evidence that increasing fiber in the diet can lower cholesterol. A specific source of fiber, psyllium (the type found in Metamucil), was shown to lower cholesterol in some patients. Other types of fiber in the diet may be helpful. Easy ways to increase the fiber in your diet to the recommended 20–35 grams per day are discussed on p. 131.

Diet to Lower Triglycerides

If triglycerides are above 250 then you can adjust your diet to lower triglycerides. This is basically a low-fat diet. If you follow the Step I diet to control cholesterol, then you will also be taking the steps needed for diet control of triglycerides. Follow the guidelines in chapter 7 for reducing fat and cholesterol in the diet and ask your doctor about any special individual needs you may have.

Can Diet or Other Steps Raise HDL Cholesterol?

Since HDL cholesterol protects against heart attack, experts suggest that the goal should be to maintain *HDL cholesterol above 60*. Exercise can help control weight, which can also help increase HDL cholesterol. Low to moderate amounts of alcohol as discussed on pp. 33–34 may help raise HDL cholesterol. If you are overweight, the greater the excess weight in the abdomen compared to the rest of the body, the lower the HDL cholesterol may be.

Dietary changes to control cholesterol may have a beneficial effect, but probably will not help if the only abnormality is low HDL cholesterol.

Stopping smoking in some studies resulted in an increase in HDL cholesterol within one month for many persons. This good effect may be even more prominent in women. Estrogen treatment in women after menopause also increases HDL cholesterol.

Regular Exercise to Control Cholesterol

A regular exercise program that includes such simple activities as walking can help lower cholesterol by helping to reduce excess weight. Regular exercise, apart from its effect on weight reduction, can *lower LDL cholesterol and triglycerides and raise HDL cholesterol,* especially in men—even after heart attack. In these patients there is evidence that the physical exercise directly helps the heart, but also helps indirectly by lowering cholesterol and delaying or arresting the atherosclerosis.

If you already have heart disease you can benefit from an exercise program guided by your doctor. Also, exercise can safely be done in a cardiac rehabilitation program.

MEDICATIONS TO CONTROL CHOLESTEROL AND TRIGLYCERIDES

Lowering LDL Cholesterol with Medication

If, despite diet, LDL cholesterol remains *over* 130 in those with other risk factors or over 100 in those who already have coronary heart disease, medications can help. Researchers have shown that if coronary heart disease is already present, reversal of the blockage is more likely if LDL cholesterol remains below 100. Some medications used to lower LDL cholesterol also have the added benefit of raising HDL cholesterol. Both of these changes are good for heart risk.

Some of the most common medications used to lower LDL cholesterol are listed in table 6.6.

Table 6.6
Some of the Most Common Medications for Controlling Cholesterol

Brand Name	Generic Name
Mevacor	Lovastatin
Zocor	Simvastatin
Questran, Questran Light	Cholestyramine
Colestid	Colestipol
Lopid	Gemfibrozil
Niacor, Nicobid, Nicolar, Slo-Niacin	Niacin and Niacin delayed-release
Pravachol	Pravastatin
Lorelco	Probucol
Lescol	Fluvastatin

Others:

Fish oil
Garlic
Estrogen

Note: Mevacor, Zocor, and Pravachol can effectively lower total cholesterol and LDL cholesterol and may raise HDL cholesterol. If you take them once each day, they should be taken in the evening to increase their effectiveness.

Patients in one study who took Mevacor were more likely to have delay or reversal of the coronary narrowing.

Occasional nausea, rash or headache can occur. Mild elevation in liver tests as measured in blood tests is also possible, so blood tests need to be done at least every few months.

Note: Lopid lowers triglycerides and can increase HDL cholesterol while lowering LDL cholesterol. The drug is usually well tolerated with only occasional nausea.

Note: Lorelco can lower total cholesterol and LDL cholesterol but can also lower HDL cholesterol. It is usully well-tolerated but can occasionally cause diarrhea.

Note: Fish oil capsules or dietary supplements containing fish such as herring can lower triglycerides; they may also lower LDL cholesterol.

Note: Niacin can lower total cholesterol, lower LDL cholesterol, and triglycerides, and raise HDL cholesterol. It is usually the least expensive of this group of medications. The most common side effect of niacin products is a flush or warm feeling accompanied by an itching sensation. This may be lessened by taking a lower dose, using delayed release niacin, taking the niacin with meals, or taking an aspirin before the niacin. Changes in vision and in blood glucose, and abnormal liver tests as measured by blood tests (especially with the delayed release niacin) can occur, so a regular checkup is needed.

Note: Garlic has been shown in some studies to lower total cholesterol, although it is not as effective as the other medications listed. See p. 101.

Note: Estrogen treatment of postmenopausal women, discussed on p. 45, can raise HDL cholesterol, and may help prevent the tendency for LDL cholesterol to increase, which happens after menopause.

The Good News: Coronary Blockages *Can Be* Reversed!

Studies have shown that patients treated with medication to lower cholesterol had more reversal of blockages and two to three times less new blockage in coronary arteries. This is important, since almost half of the heart attack patients in many hospitals are persons already known to have heart disease. Old blockages may be reversible; if new blockages could also be reduced, many "second" heart attacks might be prevented.

Some patients need more than one medication plus a diet to lower their cholesterol. Researchers have shown that in more severe cases of high cholesterol these treatment combinations can lower LDL cholesterol, raise HDL cholesterol, and can result in some reversal of the coronary blockage in over one-third of patients.

Each medication for cholesterol control has a slightly different overall effect. For example, one may mainly lower LDL cholesterol with less effect on HDL cholesterol, while another may have a greater effect on triglycerides. As we've said, the best goal in lowering your heart risk most effectively is to lower LDL cholesterol *and* raise HDL cholesterol, not simply lower the former.

Raise HDL Cholesterol

Although it is good to raise HDL cholesterol above 60, so far there is no excellent medication to raise only HDL cholesterol in cases where LDL cholesterol is already normal. Regular exercise, weight control, low to moderate amounts of alcohol, kicking the cigarette habit, and changing the types of food in your diet as discussed on p. 101 are the best ways to raise HDL cholesterol.

Lowering Triglycerides

When triglycerides remain elevated even with diet, medications may be used to lower your heart risk. Some medications that lower cholesterol can also reduce triglycerides. Of course, your heart-healthy diet should also be continued.

Not every patient responds in the same way to the medications for cholesterol control. It may take time to find the best combination to properly *lower LDL cholesterol, raise HDL cholesterol, and lower triglycerides.* Each of these is important for reducing the risk of heart attack.

Side Effects

Side effects are possible with these medications, even though most people have no problems. It is a good idea to check with your doctor to decide how often blood tests should be taken to be sure no side effects, such as those listed on p. 103, occur and to monitor your cholesterol and triglyceride levels.

Treating All Ages?

Should persons of all ages be treated with medications to control cholesterol? Since the diets described are generally healthy, they should definitely be followed, along with other nonmedication treatments, if your tests results show high LDL cholesterol or triglycerides.

Among older men and women, the risks for heart disease are not so directly related to cholesterol level. Because of this, after age seventy, medications to control cholesterol should be carefully evaluated in each case. And after age eighty, it is possible in many cases to avoid medication for cholesterol, since in tests done so far it has no definitely proven benefit. The steps for treatment without medication are still recommended and healthy.

STOP SMOKING

The risk of heart attack goes up when you smoke cigarettes. The most dangerous combinations occur when smokers are also hypertensive, have high cholesterol, or take birth control pills. The good news is that you can quickly lower your risk simply by kicking the smoking habit.

These facts are important for those who are planning to prevent heart attack altogether. But for those who have already had a heart attack, smoking poses so high a risk that it is imperative to stop.

Remember, even light smoking (one to four cigarettes per day) greatly increases the risk of heart attack in men and women. Even non-smokers who are exposed to cigarette smoke in their environment have a higher risk.

The evidence is clear: stop smoking to reduce your risk of heart attack. The most important step is to make an honest commitment to stop. This should be because you realize the risks involved as well as the major benefits in reduced heart attack and risk of death.

Most people who try to stop smoking just to please someone else find it extremely difficult to do so. It helps to look at the situation realistically: once you're convinced in your own mind, quitting does become easier. The following benefits may help convince you that it is time to make the change:

- lowered risk of heart attack and death

- lowered risk of death after coronary bypass surgery and other surgery

- lowered risk of atherosclerosis and blockage of arteries in the legs with its risk of gangrene in the feet and legs

- improved physical endurance

- reduced risk of peptic ulcers

- lowered risk of cancers of the lung, mouth, throat, esophagus, kidney, bladder, and pancreas

- reduced risk of cough, emphysema, chronic bronchitis, and other lung disease

- improved HDL cholesterol.

Some do better to stop "cold turkey." Others find it beneficial to stop gradually over days or weeks. Whichever way you choose, there is a great deal of support available. Contact your local chapter of the American Heart Association, American Lung Association or American Cancer Society for information about local programs. A reputable smoking withdrawal clinic may be helpful.

Your doctor can help you by prescribing nicotine patches or nicotine gum to help during the period of nicotine withdrawal. This period is usually most bothersome during the first two weeks. Nicotine patches or transdermal systems (Habitrol, Nicoderm, Nicotrol, and Prostep) can actually be used for about three months in gradually decreasing doses.

About 80 percent of those who use these patches can successfully kick cigarettes. The success rate increases when accompanied by a genuine personal commitment and sincere desire to stop smoking. It actually may be best to choose a time when you don't have many sources of high stress which may make stopping harder.

If necessary, other medications to control the withdrawal symptoms can be prescribed by your doctor. Support from family, friends, or a professional such as a clinical psychologist trained in this area may be helpful. The benefits of stopping cigarettes are high enough for you to go to great lengths to accomplish your goal.

EXERCISE CAN BE EASY

For prevention of heart disease, an exercise program can be easy, convenient, and enjoyable. The goal is to walk briskly twenty to thirty minutes each day or do something that has equivalent value.

The value of exercise for heart disease, excess weight, stress, and cholesterol control has already been described on p. 36. Remember that HDL cholesterol with its protective effect might be raised with as little as eight to ten miles of walking per week—only a little over one mile a day!

Check with Your Doctor

Before starting any exercise program for prevention, check with your doctor to make sure it is safe. Then walk for one to two minutes each day and gradually increase to thirty minutes of brisk walking. You can increase the time or speed of walking, but if you experience shortness of breath or chest discomfort, stop until you have talked with your physician.

Make Your Program Convenient

Your exercise should be convenient—of easy access and easy to start each day—or you probably won't continue it for months and years, as you need to for good health. This should be a complete lifestyle change, not a brief diversion! Some prefer to use a treadmill at home, a bicycle or a stationary exercise bike, swim, jog, jump rope, or a combination. Some would rather go to a gym or health club for exercise or attend an aerobic exercise class. Choose the exercise or combination of exercises you like, and start slowly. But plan to continue them permanently for your heart's sake.

If You Have Heart Disease, Proceed Cautiously

If you already have heart disease, your exercise program needs to be individualized. This is best done by your doctor or cardiologist, and will depend both on your actual ability to exercise and the amount of energy you will need for work and other activities. Estimates are that if you participate in such a program, your ability to work may improve by 25 percent.

With exercise testing on a treadmill your doctor can accurately gauge your ability for exercise. Then an exercise program that provides about 50 to 60 percent of maximum activity is begun. This is a sensible level for gradually increasing your ability to exercise and to improve the heart. At first it may be a good idea to be a part of a cardiac rehabilitation program so that you can be shown exactly how much to exercise. Remember that these exercise sessions are quite safe if they are done properly and under appropriate supervision.

Some people with heart disease may need to periodically interrupt exercise with short periods of rest or take lighter exercise. At first, exercise sessions may be very light, lasting only a few minutes. The sessions can be gradually increased in length and intensity. The formal exercise program for heart patients should continue for one to three months, after which it may be possible to continue a personal program on their own.

There is no upper age limit for people with or without heart disease with respect to these exercise programs. Physical training and conditioning have been shown to be effective at least up to age eighty. In each case, the program can be designed with the person's own abilities and safety requirements in mind.

LOSE WEIGHT

Being overweight increases heart risk as well as risks for hypertension; high blood cholesterol; high triglycerides, diabetes mellitus; cancer of the colon, rectum, and prostate in men; and cancer of the breast, uterus, ovary, and gall bladder in women. The more overweight you are, the higher the risk of death from any of these causes.

Weight loss must be a long-term plan and commitment. Ways to make it easy are discussed in chapter 7. Success is most likely if you aim for one-half to one pound weight loss weekly—this would add up to as much as fifty-two pounds in a year! This rate of weight loss is much longer lasting than a quick and faddish loss of ten to fifteen pounds in the first month. Many of us have friends who have found that fast weight loss rarely lasts.

Diet control combined with a moderate exercise program, such as walking, is the method of weight loss with the highest success rate. Make your commitment and proceed slowly to reach your goal. If you need help, talk to your doctor or a dietician and get the job done.

TAKE CARE OF THE STRESS

Stress management is important because it can let you teach yourself how to deal with and avoid stress. Try to remember that all stress is not bad, and that we can't always prevent every stress. But we *can* *control* the way we react and manage our stress.

Since stress can increase heart risk, stress management should be a part of your long-term prevention program. If you have coronary heart disease, it is even more important to manage stress well. Stress management for you may include listening to music or some other activity that produces the relaxation response as described on pp. 146ff.

Stress management can lower heart risk. Some studies show a reduction of blood pressure, resulting in fewer heart and angina attacks. The effects of such a preventive measure may be discernible within a few months. Some researchers even report fewer deaths from heart disease when stress management is added to treatment.

There are many ways to control stress and use the relaxation response. If your rate of stress is high, it would be a good idea to seek advice from a clinical psychologist or other specialist trained in stress management.

WORK ON YOUR PERSONALITY

Personality, as discussed on pp. 44–45, can play a part in heart disease, with type A behavior having been shown to cause a higher risk of heart attack. Many type A individuals are not even aware of their higher risk. Answer the questions on pp. 44–45 to see whether you fit the type A personality profile. If you do, remember that the two components of this personality most important for heart attack are: hostility and anger.

Hostility and anger can be reduced through stress management and simple instruction in behavior modification. Research shows a real benefit in changing hostility and anger; when they are reduced or eliminated, heart patients have fewer future heart problems.

This is an area in which you may benefit from the advice of a professional trained in behavior modification, such as a clinical psychologist. In any case, don't ignore this problem. If you do suffer from excess anger or hostility, simply take care of it just as you would any of the other risk factors, and enjoy the benefits of peace of mind as well as lower heart risk.

CHECK ALL RISK FACTORS AT MENOPAUSE

As discussed on p. 45, women have higher HDL cholesterol level than men beginning around the age of puberty. Then at menopause, as estrogen levels drop, HDL cholesterol also drops and LDL cholesterol rises. Both these changes create a higher heart attack risk. These are probably the major reasons for the increase in heart attack risk in women after menopause.

Estrogen Tablets Offer the Greatest Benefit

Even a small drop in HDL cholesterol can greatly increase heart risk. Much of the higher risk from estrogen loss can be corrected simply by taking estrogen supplements. Estrogen tablets are more effective for this purpose than estrogen patches or injections. Adding progestin treatments decreases the protective effect of the estrogen.

Overall, the risk of heart disease and other cardiovascular disease is reduced 40 to 50 percent in women who take estrogen after menopause. Although estrogen treatment is not recommended in every case, every woman around the time of menopause should check her risk factors, with the help and advice of her physician, and make a decision whether to use estrogen. The other benefits of estrogen include prevention of osteoporosis and control of hot flushes and other symptoms of menopause.

Estrogen's Side Effects

The side effects of estrogen include a higher chance of spotty or irregular vaginal bleeding if you have not undergone removal of your uterus (hysterectomy). This is because the estrogen stimulates the uterus just as it did before menopause.

Estrogen treatment increases the risk of cancer of the lining of the uterus (endometrial cancer). This problem can be controlled by using lower doses of estrogen and by regular checkups with your gynecologist for a simple test that samples the uterine lining (an endometrial biopsy). This is done once or twice a year for safety. Then, if a problem is detected, it can be eliminated quickly.

Estrogens may slightly increase the risk of breast cancer in women. If you are at increased risk of breast cancer already (that is, if you have already had breast cancer or some other abnormality, or have a family history of breast cancer), you should discuss this with your doctor.

CONTROL DIABETES MELLITUS

As discussed on p. 47, diabetics are two to three times more likely to suffer from coronary heart disease. The presence of hypertension and high cholesterol increases the chances even further in diabetics.

Controlling the blood glucose of diabetics is important, because poor glucose control leads to higher LDL cholesterol and higher triglycerides, which are especially common among diabetics. Good glucose control has also been shown to lower the chance of kidney disease. This is important because persons who have kidney problems resulting from diabetes, such as increased protein in the urine, run a higher risk of heart disease.

Until researchers provide specific answers to the problem of diabetes, it is important that diabetics control their blood glucose as effectively as possible, as well as each of their other risk factors.

FAMILY HISTORY: CAN WE CHANGE IT?

As discussed on p. 49, we cannot change our family history; however, we can control many of the actual risk factors that our family history bequeaths. For example, if your father died at an early age of heart attack, try to learn what risk factors were actually present: Did he smoke cigarettes? Did he have hypertension? Did he have high blood cholesterol? Focus on and control these individual risk factors. In this way, perhaps even some of our "family history" can be rewritten.

ASPIRIN HAS A PROVEN BENEFIT

Aspirin has been found to change the way platelets, cells found in the blood, act in blood vessels. This is important, since blood platelets may be involved in the development of coronary atherosclerosis. They may play a role in the tiny injuries and blood clots that begin and contribute to aterial blockage. Aspirin may prevent clots of cracks and fissues in the narrowed walls of the arteries (see chapter 2). By limiting this effect, aspirin can help reduce or slow atherosclerosis.

In studies of patients with coronary heart disease, those who took one aspirin every other day had fewer first heart attacks. Men with no known heart disease had over 40 percent fewer first heart attacks. Women over fifty years of age who took aspirin had over 30 percent fewer first heart attacks.

Among patients who have already experienced a heart attack, some studies show over 30 percent reduction in future heart attacks in those who took a low dose of aspirin.

Aspirin is commonly given in heart attack when a patient is hospitalized. Studies in these cases show a much lower risk of future heart attack and death from heart disease. This does not prevent any of the other necessary treatments for heart attack.

This beneficial effect comes from low doses of aspirin. The exact recommended dose is not yet known, but it is thought to be one aspirin or less per day or every other day. Higher doses may increase side effects in the stomach and cause other medical problems. The most common side effects noticed with steady low doses are easy bruising or bleeding and upset stomach. Your doctor will advise you about your own situation.

7

Your Heart-Healthy Diet

"You are what you eat." How many times have we heard this statement? Research has proven that many common diseases can be related to the foods we put in our bodies each day. For example, a diet high in sodium can raise blood pressure levels, while one low in complex carbohydrates, including fruits and vegetables, can adversely affect the intestinal tract. And a diet high in fat can lead to many types of cancer, obesity, and, yes, even heart attack.

The foods you eat can play a vital role in the prevention and treatment of heart attack. Diet programs have shown report after report of actual case studies of people with chronic heart disease who have made dramatic strides to health by following these heart-healthy programs. There are other diet programs that boast of healing unhealthy hearts, and the premise is the same for most: avoid heart damage and associated diseases by watching both what you eat and what you don't eat every day.

THE BAD NEWS: AMERICANS ARE TOO FAT

Statistics show that from 25 to 64 percent of Americans are overweight. For people with a history of heart attack, staying at a reasonable weight is important for reducing the chances of further heart problems. Weighing as little as ten or fifteen pounds over your desired weight can exacerbate a heart condition, elevating blood pressure and cholesterol.

What you eat also greatly affects the way you feel. If you are overweight and are recovering from heart attack or if you wish to prevent heart attack in the future, this chapter is important for you. We outline the latest dietary recommendations for heart health and weight loss. If you are not overweight and can maintain a proper weight level, then review this chapter to see if you are following the important nutritional guidelines for prevention of heart attack.

EAT FOR GOOD HEALTH

The last thing many people who have had a heart attack want to be bothered with is another schedule or program. One 62-year-old woman who has suffered two heart attacks said: "After I take my medications, do my exercise routine, then do the deep breathing for stress reduction, the last thing I want to worry about is a weight loss program." Another patient told of going on a popular low-calorie liquid diet while trying to lose weight, only to find it didn't work. While losing weight during the twelve weeks he followed the liquid diet, he gained back what he had lost, plus an additional seven pounds, as soon as he went off it.

You can take comfort in the knowledge that this chapter is not about following a liquid weight loss diet or a even a restrictive diet program. These very low calorie or food restrictive diets don't work for long-term weight control. Studies show that approximately 95 percent of those who go on weight loss diets will gain all or some of it back within one year. In fact, some studies have found that after a period of five years, not one "advertised" diet program was successful in keeping the weight off.

Instead of giving you a quick fix for weight reduction, we will encourage you to focus on eating for a healthy heart instead of eating to reduce weight. We have listed easy-to-follow guidelines recommended by the American Heart Association and the National Cholesterol Education Program for a healthy heart. We have also included the Pyramid Diet Plan advocated by the American Dietetics Association for you to follow. This gives the foods necessary for health in the proper amounts and categories. It is our greatest wish that you will *win* with heart attack, so let's start eating for a healthy heart!

GUIDELINES TO FOLLOW

1. Eat Less Than 30 Percent of Total Calories from Fat

More than 80 million people in the United States have elevated cholesterol levels and 63 million suffer from one or more forms of heart and blood vessel disease. The typical American diet, high in fat and calories until recent years, remains a major factor in the development of heart disease. The risk factors, including elevated blood cholesterol and triglycerides and obesity, are known to be closely linked to the type and amount of fat in the diet.

Reducing fat (mainly saturated fat) may be the easiest and most healthful way to reduce your weight and chances for heart attack.

A Common American Diet: High Fat

A common American diet contains more than 40 percent of its calories from fat. Since fats supply over twice as many calories per gram as carbohydrate or protein, we take in more calories, leading to weight gain. As the following table shows:

- 1 gram of fat = 9 calories

- 1 gram of carbohydrate = 4 calories

- 1 gram of protein = 4 calories.

While the American Heart Association recommends that Americans reduce their intake of fats to no more than 30 percent of total calories, most people greatly exceed that figure. Many researchers point to this high fat intake as the cause of a number of our chronic diseases, including heart attack. Think of the last time you indulged in a tender filet mignon, onion rings, and baked potato smothered in sour cream, and then followed this gastronomical delight with a piece of New York cheese cake. This meal, while certainly appealing to many of us, provides more than 50 percent of its calories from fat—and most of it is saturated!

As you begin to think heart healthy, you need to avoid the obvious high-fat foods. For example:

- Fried chicken contains 55 percent fat.

- A fast food quarter-pound hamburger contains 55 percent fat.

- A fish fillet doubles its calories when bathed in butter and fried in oil.

- Cole slaw gets over 77 percent of its calories from its fatty dressing.

You may question that last fact: After all, isn't cole slaw a salad? Yes, but while the cabbage is a wonderful heart-healthy choice containing less than .3 grams of fat, the mayonnaise or oil piles in the hidden fat with over 22 grams per serving! Even though it is a salad, cole slaw made this way is certainly not going to help your heart or weight. But you can certainly still enjoy cole slaw—made a healthier way, by using low-fat or even no-fat mayonnaise.

As you begin to change your eating habits to heal your heart, think "lower" fat. Instead of eating like a bird to do this, begin your daily menu plan with low-fat foods, including vegetables, fruits, breads, whole grain cereals, legumes, fish, and skinless chicken. These heart-healthy foods will allow you to feel full and still lose weight. Remember, some fats are actually good for the heart and should be included in your diet. We'll discuss those in a moment.

Watch for Hidden Fats

Fat can be easily recognizable in such foods as potato chips and sour cream dip, cheeseburgers and fries, and a bacon and egg breakfast. But some fats are dangerously hidden in such seemingly healthy foods as oatmeal and raisin bars, some types of peanut butter, cheese, some yogurts, popcorn cooked in oil, granola, and more. This is why everyone must become accustomed to reading labels and knowing the nutritional makeup of the foods we eat.

While the recommendation is to limit fat to less than 30 percent of the total intake of calories each day, many researchers and physicians take this one step further, and ask patients to lower fat intake to 20 to 25 percent or less of their total caloric intake each day. The *Journal of the American Medical Association* published the results of a study showing that a diet providing 30 percent of calories from fat may help prevent new arterial blockages from forming; but in persons with heart disease, it does not prevent clogged arteries from getting worse. This study recommends no more than 25 percent of total calories from fat. The success of the Pritikin Program and the very low-fat diet established by Dr. Dean Ornish is based on the proven theory of eating even less fat than is recommended, with a grand total each day of no more than 10 percent fat.

A recent study at Cornell University found that women who ate a low-fat diet lost an average of one-half pound a week while eating as much food as they wanted. These women, divided into two groups, ate either a typical diet with 37 percent of calories from fat or a 25 percent fat diet. Both groups were allowed to each as much as they wanted; the low-fat group could even eat foods like pizza and ice cream prepared with reduced-fat ingredients. The women who ate the low-fat diet lost weight without being concerned about how much they ate or counting calories.

Begin to Make Smart Choices

While staying on a low-fat or no-fat diet seems out of reach for many of us, it can be done easily by making some voluntary substitutions in our daily diet—skim milk for whole milk, reduced-fat margarine for butter, no-fat yogurt for regular yogurt, baked skinless chicken for fried chicken, and baked low-fat crackers or no-fat pretzels instead of fried chips (see the following table for more ways to reduce fat).

Table 7.1
Ways to Reduce Fat in Your Diet

Change This	To This
ice cream	ice milk, sherbet, frozen yogurt
butter	no-fat or reduced-fat margarine
whole milk	low-fat or skimmed milk
creamed soups	low-fat variety prepared with skimmed milk
french fries	baked oven fries
potato chips	baked crackers or pretzels
cream	evaporated skim milk
fried chicken	baked chicken without skin
spaghetti sauce with meat	tomato sauce
hamburger	chicken sandwich
candy bar	fudgsicle
grilled cheese sandwich	grilled cheese with no-fat cheese
chocolate candy	no-fat jelly beans or candy corn
omelet	egg substitutes or egg whites
pancakes, biscuits, muffins	bagels, English muffins, rice cakes
chocolate chip cookies	fig bars, gingersnaps
pound cake	angel food cake
regular mayonnaise	low-fat or no-fat mayonnaise
tartar sauce	cocktail sauce or salsa
cream cheese on bagel	no-fat cream cheese on bagel

Read Your Labels

How do you know if a product is high or low in fat? *Read the label!* Package labels include the ingredients, the calories, the nutrients, the sodium, and much more for the consumer's information (see table 7.2 for a sample label).

Table 7.2. Sample Label

Clam Chowder

Ingredients: Clam broth, potatoes, tomato paste, carrots, clams, celery, sweet peppers, modified food starch, salt, vegetable oil (corn, cottonseed, or partially hydrogenated soybean oil), water, wheat flour, monosodium glutamate, dehydrated parsley, natural flavoring, yeast extract, and spice.

Nutritional Information Per Serving

Serving size:	4 oz.
Servings per container:	2¾
Calories:	70
Protein (grams):	2
Carbohydrate (grams):	10
Fat (grams):	2
Cholesterol:	less than 5 mg/serving
Sodium:	820 mg/serving

After reading the label, you can figure out whether this is a high-, moderate-, or low-fat food by using the following formula:

1 gram fat = 9 calories
If the serving has 2 grams of fat, then
$2 \times 9 = 18$ calories from fat.
If the total calories of the serving are 70, then:
$18/70 = 25.7\%$ of calories from fat.

This would be considered a low-fat food with under 26 percent of fat calories.

Calculating Fat Calories

Trying to stay below 30 percent or an even more healthful 20 percent of fat calories from fat each day means that you must carefully calculate this amount. After several weeks of doing this, it will become a "low-fat habit," and you will naturally turn to the healthier foods instead of unhealthy fat choices.

If you eat 1500 calories each day, you can calculate your fat calories by using the following formula:

1500 calories × 30 percent fat calories = 450 calories from fat.

You can now determine how many grams of fat allowed per day:

450 calories from fat / 9 calories per gram of fat = 50 grams of fat per day.

Table 7.3
Fat Content of Selected Foods
(By Percentage of Calories from Fat)

Foods with less than 30% fat

Angel food cake
Bread
Chicken (roasted, light meat without skin)
Cod fillets (broiled)
Cottage cheese (1% fat)
Crab (cooked)
Crackers (saltines)
Dried beans, lentils, and peas (cooked without fat)
Fruits, all (with exceptions listed)
Halibut fillets (broiled)
Ice milk (vanilla)
Milk (1% fat)
Pasta
Popcorn (plain)
Pretzels
Rice
Sherbet (orange)
Shrimp (steamed, shelled)
Skim milk
Tuna (white [albacore] canned in water)
Turkey (roasted, light meat without skin)
Yogurt (plain, low-fat)
Yogurt (fruit flavor, low-fat)
Yogurt (frozen)
Vegetables, all (with exceptions listed)
Wheat germ

Foods with 30% to 40% fat

Beef (rump lean only)
Brownie (from mix)
Cottage cheese (creamed [4% fat])
Flounder (fried)
Flank steak
Granola
Ice milk (chocolate)
Milk (2% fat)
Shrimp (fried)
Turkey (roasted, dark meat without skin)

Table 7.3 (cont'd.)

Foods with 40% to 50% fat

Chicken (roasted dark meat without skin)
Chicken (roasted, light meat with skin)
Cookies (chocolate chip)
Crackers (butter type)
Cupcake with icing
Ice cream (vanilla)
Milk (whole)
Pork loin (lean roasted)
Salmon (canned)
Tuna (white [albacore] canned in oil)
Yogurt (whole milk)

Foods with 50% or more fat

Avocado
Bacon
Beef rump roast (marbled)
Bologna
Butter
Cheeses (hard such as cheddar, Swiss)
Chicken (roasted, dark meat with skin)
Coconut
Coffee creamer palm oil (dry powder)
Cream cheese
Cream (half and half)
Cream (table)
Doughnut (cake-type)
Doughnut (raised)
Egg
Frankfurters
Ground beef
Margarine
Peanuts (roasted)
Peanut butter
Pork loin (lean and fat)
Salami
Sausage pork
Sour cream

Fat Grams

Calories Per Day	Grams of Fat 30% of calories	Grams of Fat 20% of calories
1000	33 grams	20 grams
1200	40 grams	24 grams
1500	50 grams	30 grams
1800	60 grams	36 grams
2000	67 grams	40 grams
2200	73 grams	44 grams
2400	87 grams	48 grams

Guidelines to Reduce Fat

The more serious you are about controlling fat in your diet, the more closely you may want to follow these guidelines:

Keep Close Watch on the Fat in Your Diet

- Keep your fat intake to 30 percent or less of your daily caloric intake. You can easily do this by purchasing *only* no-fat or low-fat items. Why put temptation in front of you?

- Stay away from foods high in saturated fats (no more than 10 percent of your total calories per day).

- Choose your fats wisely. *No more* than 10 percent of your calories should come from polyunsaturated fat. Ten to 15 percent of your calories should come from monounsaturated fat found in olive oil (see the Mediterranean Diet on p. 33).

- Invest in a pocket-sized fat gram counter, and use it to look up the fat content of foods you regularly eat. Zero in on the highest fat foods and make some changes you can live with.

- Make subtle changes each week. Switching to skim milk instead of whole milk and eating skinless baked chicken instead of fried chicken could result in a reduction of calories—enough to lose 10 pounds in one year!

Take Advantage of Carbohydrates to Fill Up, Not Out

- Fill up on complex carbohydrates (starch and fiber) by eating at least five servings of fruits and vegetables per day instead of making high-fat choices. But be careful with carbohydrates: a low-fat, high-carbo-hydrate diet is a sensible way to eat, but it's not a license for gluttony. Even complex carbohydrates will put weight on you if eaten in excess. Show moderation.

- When choosing vegetables, turn down those with cheesy sauces and turn instead to raw or sauteed vegetables.

- Go slow on prepared cole slaw, potato salad, macaroni salad, and pasta salad. These are all high in fat *unless* they are made with no-fat or low-fat dressings. Opt for the low-fat or no-fat salad dressings on your green salad, or use flavored vinegars (no fat or calories!) and leave off the oil.

What about Meat Choices?

- Choose fish, skinned poultry, and lean red meat. Be sure to trim all visible fat from meat and poultry before cooking. When selecting cuts of meat, choose the "skinniest" cuts of top round, tip round, sirloin and chuck.

- Buy ground beef that is at least 90 percent lean or choose ground round or ground sirloin.

- Exchange ground turkey or chicken for half or even all the beef in a recipe for spaghetti, chili, meat loaf, or burgers. (Read the labels and buy ground white turkey or chicken, which has half the fat of dark meat).

- Instead of frying meats, broil, bake, grill, steam, or sauté meats (fish and chicken) in defatted broth.

- There is a breakfast meat that is not high in fat! Choose Canadian bacon with only one gram of fat.

- Avoid self-basting turkeys which are injected with heavy oils. Instead, use olive oil and defatted chicken or turkey broth for preparing a turkey.

- Buy water-packed tuna and save on fat calories while getting much-needed omega-3s.

Beans Are Good for Your Heart!

- Learn how to use tofu and legumes as meat substitutes. Have several "meatless" high-protein meals each week by combining lentils (red beans, navy beans, and Great Northern beans being just a few examples) with pasta or rice. This meal will fill you up and is very low in fat.

- Use vegetarian refried beans in your tacos instead of meat filling. Make sure you check the label for the no-fat or low-fat variety.

- Add low-fat ground turkey to red beans to make chili, or use beans instead of meat for spaghetti sauces.

Avoid Adding "Extras" to Your Meal

- When choosing dairy products—go for the skimmed! Choose low-fat or no-fat cheeses, including cottage cheese, sour cream, cream cheese, yogurt, skim milk, ice milk, sherbet, frozen yogurt, and sorbet. Also, skim the broth for soups using defatted liquids. Canned undiluted skim milk for cream soups makes an excellent low-fat choice for mealtime.

- Instead of using a whole egg in a recipe, use two egg whites or egg substitute (¼ cup = one egg).

- Make fat-free whipped cream to top your favorite berries using chilled and whipped canned skim milk. (Add one tablespoon lemon juice and three tablespoons sugar, beat until stiff).

Choose Tasty Low-Fat Snacks

- Air-popped popcorn and rice cakes make tasty fat-free snacks. Pretzels usually have one gram of fat per ounce (check label). This low-fat snack food contains ten times less fat than potato chips.

- Use natural peanut butter with no oil or sugar added. Most grocery stores now carry peanut butter with less fat. Check your supermarket shelves.

- Animal crackers, vanilla wafers, graham crackers, and ginger snaps are all low-fat choices for cookies. But be careful here: the calories and fats add up *if* you eat too many!

- Use apple sauce, prune puree, or other fruit substitute for butter or oil in loaf cakes or drop cookies.

Don't Let Dining Out Be Your Dieting Downfall!

- Watch the hidden calories in fast foods! The calories contained in that juicy hamburger are over 50 percent fat. Also be alert for high-fat menu terms such as "creamed," "sauteed," "au gratin," and "smothered."

- When ordering a main dish, request baked or broiled chicken or beef, and remember: "extra crispy" means extra calories!

- Instead of fries, choose a baked potato. But watch your toppings! They can be loaded with fat and calories, so heap on the tomatoes, mushrooms, broccoli, carrots, and cauliflower. Leave those high-fat toppings off of pizza, and substitute onions, mushrooms, bell pepper, broccoli, and other vegetable toppings.

- Replace breakfast sandwiches with low-fat muffins or cereal.

- Try a reduced-fat milk shake or even a frozen yogurt shake over a high-fat, creamy shake.

- Skip guacamole, sour cream, and refried beans when ordering Mexican foods. Choose tacos, tostados, or corn tortilla. A taco salad in a large fried shell contains over 900 calories, and most of this is fat. See the suggestions on p. 32 for good fast food choices.

Never Say Diet Again!

Never say "diet" again. Get excited about your new, heart-healthy, low fat way of eating. Try not to refrain too much from eating the foods you enjoy. Even if you're counting fat grams, don't get too hung up on what you eat at any one meal. What's most important is how many you eat over a period of time.

2. Eat Less Than 10 Percent of Total Calories from Saturated Fat

Fats are the most concentrated source of food energy, supplying nine calories per gram, while carbohydrates and proteins have only four calories per gram. Studies have proven that a diet high in fat may increase a person's chance of obesity, which contributes to heart attack and other diseases. However, some fats are actually beneficial.

Table 7.4
Know Your Fats

A fat is a fat. True? Not at all! Fats fall into three main categories: saturated, monounsaturated, and polyunsaturated.

Saturated fat: fat that comes from animal and whole milk dairy products. This also comes from some oils. (Examples include: red meat, butter, cheeses, luncheon meats, cocoa butter, coconut oil, palm oil, cream). It is wise to limit your saturated fatty foods and try to substitute whenever possible.

Monounsaturated fat: fat that comes from plant foods, including canola and olive oils. New research suggests that these fats may actually reduce your blood cholesterol level and your risk of cardiovascular disease.

Polyunsaturated fat: fat that is found in plants, including sunflower, corn, soybean, and safflower oils. Polyunsaturated fats also can reduce blood cholesterol levels.

Table 7.5
Know Your Oils

This table lists the most common oils and what percentage of each is saturated, monounsaturated, and polyunsaturated fat. Choose oils high in monounsaturated and polyunsaturated fats, and stay away from oils high in saturated fats.

	Saturated	*Monounsaturated*	*Polyunsaturated*
Safflower oil	9	13	78
Sunflower oil	11	20	69
Corn oil	13	25	62
Olive oil	14	77	9
Soybean oil	15	24	61
Peanut oil	18	48	34
Cottonseed oil	27	19	54
Lard	41	47	12
Palm oil	51	39	10
Beef tallow	52	44	4
Butterfat	66	30	4
Palm kernel oil	86	12	2
Coconut oil	92	6	2

Eat Omega-3 Fatty Acids

Eating fish may help your heart. Studies of Eskimos' diet show that mackerel, bluefish, tuna, herring, anchovies, sardines, and salmon are high in omega-3 fatty acids, which have been shown to reduce the "bad" LDL cholesterol and raise the "good" HDL cholesterol. The Eskimos under study were found to have low levels of cholesterol, triglycerides, LDL cholesterol, and high levels of HDL cholesterol.

Guidelines have not been established regarding supplements of fish oil. You can add omega-3 fish to your diet naturally or use supplements available at health food stores or pharmacies.

When choosing healthful fish for meals, select one of the following: anchovies, bluefish, capelin, dogfish, herring, mackerel, salmon, sardines, shad, sturgeon, tuna, or whitefish.

3. Eat Less Than 300 Milligrams of Cholesterol per Day

Studies show that as many as 80 percent of middle-aged American men have cholesterol levels that place them at increased risk for heart attack. The higher the level of cholesterol, the higher the risk becomes. Cholesterol level can be directly affected by cholesterol in the diet; therefore, by lowering your blood cholesterol level, you dramatically reduce your risk of cardiovascular heart disease.

Dietary cholesterol is found in animal foods: meats, poultry, fish, egg yolks, milk, cream, cheese, butter, and other dairy foods.

Table 7.6
Cholesterol Content of Selected Foods

	Amount	*Milligrams*
Dairy		
Butter	1 tsp.	11
Margarine	1 tsp.	0
Skim milk	1 cup.	5
1%	1 cup	10
2%	1 cup	18
Whole milk	1 cup	34
Sherbet	½ cup	7
Ice cream	½ cup	30
Cream	1 tbsp.	20
Half and half	1 tbsp.	6
American cheese	1 oz.	16
Cheddar cheese	1 oz.	30
Mozzarella, part skim	1 oz.	15
Swiss cheese	1 oz.	26
Cottage cheese (1% fat)	1 cup	10
Poultry		
Chicken, dark (no skin)	3 oz.	81
Chicken, white (no skin)	3 oz.	72
Turkey, dark (no skin)	3 oz.	87
Turkey, white (no skin)	3 oz.	66

Table 7.6 (cont'd.)

	Amount	*Milligrams*
Red meat		
Bacon	1 slice	5
Beef, lean	3 oz.	78
Frankfurter	1.6 oz.	45
Ham (boiled)	3 oz.	75
Pork (lean)	3 oz.	75
Veal (lean)	3 oz.	84
Seafood/fish		
Crab	3 oz.	85
Flounder	3 oz.	70
Haddock	3 oz.	40
Lobster	3 oz.	70
Oysters	3 oz.	42
Shrimp	3 oz.	128
Tuna	3 oz.	55
Breads/Cereals/Grains		
Bread	1 slice	0
Bagel	1 whole	0
Doughnut, yeast	1	21
Oatmeal	½ cup	0
Rice (plain)	½ cup	0
Cookie (plain)	1	1
Fruits/Vegetables		
Potato (baked)	1 small	0
Potato (fried)	10 strips	0
Cabbage	½ cup	0
Apple	1 medium	0
Banana	1 medium	0

Table 7.6 (contd.)

	Amount	*Milligrams*
Miscellaneous		
Cereal		0
Egg noodles	1 cup	50
Egg whites		0
Egg yolk	1 large	272
Fruits		0
Nuts		0
Vegetables		0

4. Take in Fewer Than 3000 Milligrams a Day of Sodium

According to a United States Department of Agriculture (USDA) survey, the average American consumes a whopping 6600 mg of sodium each day. That is the amount of salt in one tablespoon, but it is two and a half times the recommended daily maximum of 2400 mg. The facts about sodium and the American way of life are startling:

- 80 percent of Americans' sodium intake comes from processed foods.

- Too much sodium can increase fluid retention and elevate blood pressure in people who are sodium sensitive.

- Many persons with hypertension could lower their blood pressure by limiting sodium.

The body's actual need for salt is only about one-half to one-and-one-half teaspoons of salt per day (1100 to 3300 mg sodium). Since many of us consume more than the daily recommended amount of salt, our bodies' needs grow subsequently less. With an estimated 50 to 60 million Americans suffering from high blood pressure, reducing the amount of salt in the diet could help some people avoid this ailment.

Although the words "salt" and "sodium" are often used interchangeably, they are not the same. Ordinary table salt is only 40 percent sodium. Many foods naturally contain sodium, including such animal products as meat, fish, poultry, milk and eggs. Vegetable products are naturally low in sodium. Most of the sodium in our diets, however, comes from commercially processed foods such as cured meats like bacon and ham, luncheon meats, sausage, frozen breaded meats, fish and seafood, and canned meats. Condiments like catsup, mustard, and steak sauce are also high in sodium. Fast foods such as hamburgers, french fries, and prepare-at-home fast foods like frozen pizza, hot dogs, sausage, creamed chipped beef, and broccoli with cheese sauce are very high in sodium. Start reading the list of ingredients on the package label to determine the sodium content, and make it a point to stay within recommended limits.

Words that include soda, sodium, or "NA" indicate sodium as a part of a preservative or flavoring agent. Some examples are monosodium glutamate, baking soda, sodium nitrate, sodium propionate, and sodium benzoate.

The U.S. Food and Drug Administration requires nutrient labels on food packages to list the sodium content. Terms such as "low sodium" and "sodium free" are also standardized to help the conscientious consumer. See the example below:

Sodium-free	Less than 5 mg sodium/serving
Very low sodium	35 mg or less sodium/serving
Low sodium	140 mg or less sodium/serving
Reduced sodium	Sodium reduced 75% compared to the product it is replacing
Unsalted, no salt added	Sodium has not been used in processing

Remember, sodium is measured in grams and milligrams. A gram is a unit of weight. There are about 28 grams in one ounce. One gram equals 1000 milligrams. The American Heart Association recommends no more than 1000 to 3000 milligrams sodium per day.

Table 7.7
Sodium Content of Selected Foods

Food	Amount	Milligrams
American cheese	1 oz.	400
Bacon	2 slices	200
Baking powder	1 tsp.	339
Baking soda	1 tsp.	821
Beans (green)	½ cup	230
Beef broth	1 cube	1150
Beef (lean)	3 oz. cooked	55
Bread	1 slice	150
Biscuit	1 (2″ diameter)	220

Table 7.7 (cont'd)

Food	Amount	Milligrams
Buttermilk	1 cup	330
Cereal (dry, flake)	⅔ cup	200
Cheeseburger (fast food)	¼ lb.	1200
Chicken noodle soup	1 cup	1100
Cornbread	1 small square	260
Cheese (cheddar)	1 oz.	200
Chocolate shake	1 average	300
Cottage cheese	4 oz.	450
Frankfurter	1½ oz.	500
Garlic powder	1 tsp.	1
Garlic salt	1 tsp.	1850
Ham	3 oz.	1000
Ketchup	1 tbsp.	156
Lite salt	¼ tsp.	250
Luncheon meat	1 slice	575
Mayonnaise	1 tbsp.	80
Meat tenderizer	1 tsp.	1750
MSG (flavor enhancer)	¾ tsp.	50
Mozzarella (part-skim)	1 oz.	132
Mustard	1 tsp.	65
Oatmeal (instant)	¾ cup	240
Oatmeal (cooked)	¾ cup	1
Olives (green)	3	720
Onion powder	1 tsp.	1
Onion salt	1 tsp.	1620
Peas (canned)	1 cup	493
Peas (frozen)	1 cup	150
Potato (boiled)	1 cup	7
Potato (instant)	1 cup	475
Potato chips	1 oz.	300
Peanut butter	1 tbsp.	100
Sauerkraut	⅔ cup	740
Sausage (pork)	2 links	380
Salt	¼ tsp.	500
Soy sauce	1 tbsp.	1030
Tomato juice	½ cup	210

Beware of:

- Canned and dried soups

- Canned vegetables

- Canned meats (tuna, chicken, etc.)

- Ketchup, mustard; barbeque, steak, and soy sauces

- Salty snack foods (potato chips, nuts, etc.)

- Luncheon meats and packaged foods

- Olives and pickles

- Bacon, cured meats, ham

- Cheese and cheese products

- Fast foods (french fries, onion rings, hamburgers, Chinese takeout)

5. Fill Your Plate with Healthful Minerals

Potassium and calcium are important for heart health. Foods such as potatoes, cantaloupe, oranges, raisins, and bananas contain potassium. Low fat dairy products contain calcium, and can be a important part of your daily diet as you work to lower blood pressure and other cardiac risk factors.

6. Eat 50 to 55 Percent of Calories from Carbohydrates

Remember when people on diets were told *not* to eat bread or pasta? Research has confirmed that these complex carbohydrates including bread, cereal, pasta, and starchy vegetables are important for a heart-healthy, low-fat diet. Fiber and complex carbohydrates are said to be nature's "miracle" foods: Not only do complex carbohydrates fill us up so we don't indulge on high fat snacks, the fiber keeps our system running smooth and regular. Research has shown that people who eat a diet high in fiber have a lower incidence of colon cancer. While the National Cancer Institute recommends eating 20 to 35 grams of fiber each day, the average person eats less than 15 grams.

There are different types of fiber: *Soluble fiber,* found in oats, fruits, vegetables, and legumes, may help to lower blood cholesterol. *Insoluble fiber,* found in wheats, bran, and whole grains, is good for the digestive system and may offer protection against certain cancers.

The Winner: Soluble Fiber

For a healthy heart, soluble fiber is the best choice. This is the type of fiber that dissolves in water (see table 7.8 below). Studies show that soluble fiber, by reducing cholesterol levels, can help keep the heart healthy.

Table 7.8
Foods High in Soluble Fiber

Acorn squash	Carrots	Peas
Apples	Cauliflower	Prunes
Baked potatoes	Citrus fruits	Pumpkin
Blueberries	Dates	Raspberries
Broccoli	Dried beans	Strawberries
Cabbage	Lentils	Sweet potatoes

You can increase your dietary fiber by including at least six servings per day of breads, cereals, pasta, rice, dried peas, and beans; two to four servings of fresh, frozen, canned, or dried fruits; and three to five servings of vegetables. As you begin to choose low-fat, high-complex carbohydrate foods for your diet, you can gradually notice a reduction in your weight. For most people with heart problems, this is an appreciated added benefit, since it helps you reduce another of the risk factors— obesity—as well as cholesterol, and you will feel better (see table 7.9 for the fiber content of some common foods).

Table 7.9
Fiber Content of Selected Foods

	Amount	*Grams*
Breads		
Bran muffin	1 average	3
Pumpernickel	1 slice	2
Rye	1 slice	2
White	1 slice	1
Whole wheat	1 slice	2

Table 7.9 (cont'd.)

	Amount	*Grams*
Cereals		
Cream of wheat, instant	1 oz.	1
Cheerios®	1 oz.	2
Fiber One®	1 oz.	12
Grits, uncooked	¼ cup	4.8
All Bran®	1 oz.	9
All Bran® with extra fiber	1 oz.	14
Bran flakes	1 oz.	4
Corn flakes	1 oz.	1
100% Bran	1 oz.	10
Oat bran	1 oz.	4
Oats (uncooked, rolled)	½ cup	4.5
Raisin Bran	1 oz.	3.5
Grape Nuts®	1 oz.	2
Dried fruits		
Dates (medium)	2½	1.5
Figs (medium)	1½	4.5
Prunes (medium)	3	4
Raisins	2 tbsp.	1.2
Fruits		
Apple (with skin)	1 medium	3
Banana	1 medium	1.5
Cantaloupe (cubes)	1 cup	2
Cherries (raw)	12	1
Grapefruit	½ medium	2.5
Grapes	15	.5
Orange	1 medium	2
Peach (raw)	1 medium	1.5
Pear (raw)	1 medium	2.8
Plum (raw)	2 small	1.5
Strawberries (raw)	1¼ cup	6.5
Tangerine	1 medium	2
Watermelon (cubes)	1¼ cup	1.75

Table 7.9 (contd.)

	Amount	*Grams*
Vegetables		
Beans (green)	½ cup	1.5
Beets (cooked)	½ cup	1.6
Broccoli (cooked)	½ cup	1.1
Cabbage (cooked)	½ cup	1.5
Carrots (cooked)	½ cup	1.4
Carrots (raw)	1 medium	3.7
Cauliflower (cooked)	½ cup	1.2
Cauliflower (raw)	1 cup	1.8
Corn (kernel)	½ cup	3.2
Kale (cooked)	½ cup	2
Kidney beans (cooked)	½ cup	7
Lettuce	1 cup	1
Peas (cooked)	½ cup	4
Potato with skin (baked)	1	3.5
Spinach (raw)	½ cup	2
Summer squash	½ cup	2.2

Guidelines to Increase Fiber

- Eat more legumes. They are very high in fiber. Red beans, black beans, Great Northern beans, and other legumes are high in fiber and have no fat. (Don't cook these with animal fat!)

- Eat raw vegetables for snacks. Two carrots will give you a day's supply of vitamin A and provide over seven grams of fiber.

- Read your cereal box at the grocery. If the cereal has no fiber or less than three grams, it probably has little nutrient value.

- Add dried fruits to your cereal. Three prunes can give you four grams of fiber.

- Keep your vegetables crisp when you cook them instead of soft. Eat these with skins on to add to the fiber content.

7. Control Total Calories to Reach and Maintain Desirable Body Weight

Statistics show that being overweight increases your risk of coronary heart disease, hypertension, high blood cholesterol, and other problems.

Some researchers have found hypertension to be almost three times higher in overweight persons than in others. The rate of diabetes mellitus was almost three times higher in overweight persons in one study. Hypertension and diabetes mellitus are definite risk factors for coronary heart disease.

See table 2.8 for desirable or ideal body weight. Check where you are for body height, weight, and build. If your body weight is 20 percent or more above the desirable weight, then you should consider a weight loss program. If you weigh 100 pounds or more above the desirable limit, your situation is extremely serious and weight loss is vital.

Experts tell us that reducing weight to desirable levels should be considered even if you are less than 20 percent overweight or if certain diseases are also present, including diabetes mellitus, hypertension, abnormal cholesterol, and high blood triglycerides. (Many specialists would also suggest weight loss for those with coronary heart disease, emphysema and chronic bronchitis, and arthritis in the hips, knees and spine.)

If you are 20 percent or more overweight, talk with your physician and make plans to begin a reasonable weight loss program safely. A reasonable diet combined with a regular exercise program is usually successful and can be painless. Before beginning a diet and exercise program, however, you must be sure that it is safe for you (see guidelines for measuring your weight loss program on pp. 138ff.). If other medical problems are present, they may affect the rate and success of your weight loss.

Now Let's Weigh In

Perhaps you have avoided height/weight charts in the past. One 50-year-old man who had a heart attack three years ago said he would never weigh himself again because he didn't weigh the same as he did in college. Remember, charts give only what is "average" for most people. These averages allow for women to be "smaller boned" than men. But if you are a small-boned male or a large-boned female, you may be normal at either end of the scale given for your height and age. It is a waste of energy to try to have the same weight that you did in high school! However, even though you cannot change your genetic makeup, you can change the way you eat.

The height/weight chart (table 2.8) gives an average weight range for all adults and takes into consideration age, height, and bone structure. The reason for including all these variables is that the new government guidelines have broader limits than before.

If you weigh slightly more than what is suggested in the height/ weight table, all you might do to feel your best is to watch your fat and caloric intake more closely, and add some exercise. But if your weight is a great deal higher than recommended, perhaps you should make some careful lifestyle and dietary changes.

GETTING STARTED WITH WEIGHT LOSS

The American Dietetic Association recommends a calorie level of no less than ten times your desired weight, with women getting at least 1200 calories and men getting at least 1400 calories per day. For example, if your goal is to be 140 pounds you should eat around 1400 calories per day. If your goal is 170 pounds, follow a daily diet of 1700 calories. If you follow this recommendation, don't expect to see a quick reduction of weight, but studies show that the chances of keeping weight off over the long term are much greater.

Nick V., a 38-year-old man with a history of heart disease in his family, wanted to lose thirty pounds with a weight goal of 140. He told of staying on a low-fat, high-complex-carbohydrate diet for six weeks, and even began a light walking and aerobics program. Still, six weeks later, Nick had gained two pounds instead of losing weight. Finally, his dietitian asked Nick to record his daily food intake for two weeks, and come in again.

After two weeks, Nick brought in a record of what he had been eating. Instead of staying about 1400 calories, Nick had eaten over 2400 calories. The choices he had made were low-fat and high complex carbohydrates, but he had eaten more calories than his body needed for weight loss. After starting over recording his daily food intake, Nick could see where he had overindulged, and began cutting back while continuing his walking and exercise program. In three months, Nick had lost twenty pounds and had changed his eating lifestyle so that the low-fat, high-complex-carbohydrate dietary changes were natural. The benefits to him of a slimmer waistline, more energy, and reduced risk of heart attack gave Nick the motivation he needed to continue his healthy new style of eating and exercise.

Keep a Food Diary

As you start a lifestyle plan of eating for a healthy heart, keeping a food diary is important. Studies have shown that when obese people who say they maintain a low-fat, low-calorie diet are asked to record their daily food intake, the results are surprising. The same people who said they ate no more than 1100 calories per day with 20 percent being fat calories, topped off at an average of over 2000 calories and with 60 percent fat calories per day. This made a tremendous difference that resulted in weight gain instead of loss!

Keeping a food diary helps you know exactly where you stand nutritionally. You may think you are eating a low-fat diet; but after calculating your fats at the end of the day, you find that you have eaten over 40 percent in fat calories. Or you may think you are getting between 20 and 35 grams of fiber each day, when, in fact, you are only getting 9 grams.

Until you get into the "heart-healthy habit," keeping a food diary will help you stay organized and honest! Use it as you would a check book, putting your daily calories, and fat and fiber grams in the spaces indicated. As you go through the day, calculate the amount of nutrients and calories in your diet. If you are over the recommended amount in calories and fats, make adjustments the next day. The diary is a good indicator of what you really eat.

Use the Food Guide Pyramid

The U.S. Department of Agriculture has designed the new Food Guide Pyramid as an excellent guideline for calculating a healthy diet (see figure 7.1). As you follow the Pyramid plan, choose most of your food choices from the wide bottom part of the pyramid and use the top part of the Pyramid only sparingly.

Be Wary of Advertised Weight Loss Programs

Even after trying to follow the pyramid plan for food choices, many people still have difficulty changing their lifestyle. Years of bad habits creep up and take over during weak moments. Some people even pay high fees to popular diet programs in order to guarantee weight loss. If you do choose a highly promoted weight loss plan, make sure you show your physician the actual plan and seek professional advice before you pay any money.

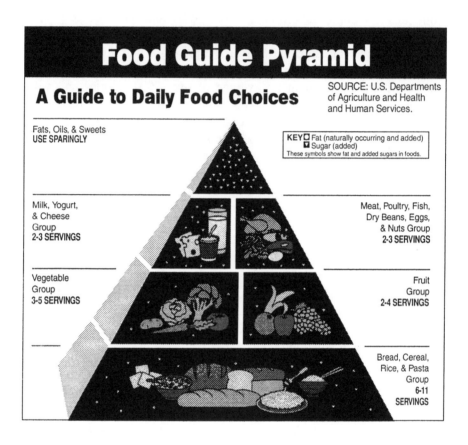

Figure 7.1
The Food Guide Pyramid: A Guide to Daily Food Choices

If you question whether a diet program is up to par, use the following checklist to determine whether the claims are healthy facts or fleeting fads.

1. Does the weight loss diet promote eating that excludes an entire food group or require you to consume only one kind of food?

Any program that completely excludes one entire food group leaves open the possibility that some vitamins and minerals essential for health may be left out. For example, some of the diet programs eliminate milk and milk products completely for weeks at a time. Other diet programs limit animal protein sources like poultry, fish, and beef. In these diets you must be more careful to ensure proper protein intake from other sources, such as breads or dairy products. This will allow you to avoid protein deficiency, which can be harmful to your body.

Be suspicious of weight loss programs that do not provide a minimum of 50 to 60 grams of protein from food sources. (The recommended daily dietary allowance for adult women is 44 grams of protein per day.)

Table 7.10

Sources of Protein	Grams
1 oz. meat, poultry, fish, cheese	7
1 egg	7
1 cup milk	8
1 serving bread or starch	3
½ cup beans or peas	6
½ cup of most other vegetables	2
1 serving fruit	0
1 tsp. fat-like oil or margarine	0

When a diet proclaims the incredible power of one particular food in promoting weight loss, be wary! This is merely the power to bore. Anyone will become tired of eating if there is only one food to eat. This may not be so bad while you are dieting, but the weight returns once you resume your old eating patterns. Too often diets that concentrate on one particular food are not providing the forty essential nutrients needed from various food groups to stay healthy.

2. Does the diet recommend very low calorie levels (less than 800 calories per day)?

When you take in less than 800 calories per day, the protein in your diet is often severely restricted. Consequently, your body may use protein from lean muscle and major vital organs to produce the energy it needs. Diets so low in calories often don't provide all the vitamins and minerals necessary to maintain health.

If the low-calorie diet is high in protein and restricted in carbohydrates from fruits, breads, and cereal, it may cause a condition called *ketosis,* which results from abnormal breakdown of fat in the body and is characterized by high levels of ketones in the blood. Ketones are substances chemically related to acetone (found in solvents such as nail polish remover). Ketogenic diets can be dangerous, especially to people with diabetes and heart, liver, or kidney disease, or dehydration.

Another hazard of such restricted calorie diets is that the dramatic weight loss is often due to water loss. This can disrupt the body's water balance and might result in an irregular heartbeat.

Finally, consuming a very low-calorie diet can lower your metabolic rate. As your body adapts to the low-calorie level, you require fewer calories to keep going, without weight loss. You also feel sluggish and worn out.

3. Does this diet promise dramatic weight loss in a short period of time? Are the results too good to be true?

When a weight loss plan advertises a weight loss of more than two to three pounds per week, beware! Any diet promoting a greater weight reduction is playing games with water loss. Rapid weight loss also causes the breakdown of muscle as well as fat, which can be harmful to the dieter.

4. Does the diet promote the special power of vitamin/mineral supplements or health foods in weight loss?

Although there are about forty vitamins and minerals essential to maintaining good health, *not one* has the dramatic power to promote weight loss. In fact, a sensible weight-loss program can provide these nutrients without expensive supplements. Health foods do not possess any special power to reduce weight either, so save your money!

5. Does the promoter of the program diet list impressive titles, degrees, credentials, or positions in associations that you never heard of?

To check the credentials of someone promoting a questionable weight loss diet, visit your library. Refer to the *Directory of Colleges and Universities* to determine whether health care promoters hold degrees from an accredited institution. You can also check the legitimacy of their professional organizations in the *Encyclopedia of Associations*. Finally, ask your doctor for a recommendation or see a registered dietician. These professionals are trained to know which diets are gimmicks and which will work—safely.

WEIGHING YOUR DIET PROGRAM

The checklist below will help you determine whether a weight loss program is sound and suitable for you.

- The program has a comprehensive approach: weight loss, diet, exercise, and lifestyle change.

- The diet promises gradual and steady weight loss (one-half to one pound per week).

- The food choices include about 20 percent of total calories as protein (fish, chicken, lean beef).

- The menu plan includes about 50 percent of total calories from carbohydrates (bread, cereal, fruit).

- The diet is adaptable to your lifestyle, taking into consideration your home and work situation, and personal tastes.

- The plan has a maintenance program to help you keep your weight off.

- The program teaches you how to prepare nutritious, reduced calorie meals.

- The frequency of visits meets your needs.

- There is an attempt to enlist family support through training.

- The staff has the necessary educational and professional backgrounds to run a weight loss program.

- The program, including special foods or supplements, is affordable.

The Mediterranean Diet

There are many factors to look at when considering the Mediterranean Diet, already described. It uses plenty of olive oil, which is full of cholesterol-cutting monounsaturated fats; but it is also rich in fruits and vegetables and low in meat. So before you simply take the bottle of olive oil and pour it over your food, keep the total picture in mind. See p. 33 for more information on how the Mediterranean Diet can reduce risks for heart attack.

What about Nuts?

As discussed on p. 34, studies have shown that nuts high in mono-unsaturated fat may have beneficial effects on the heart. Walnuts and almonds have been touted for their LDL cholesterol-lowering qualities. Many studies have shown that Seventh Day Adventists who eat nuts have a lower rate of heart attack. Nuts are also high in calories, so if you are on a weight reduction program to help your heart, add this high fat food in moderation and stay within your calorie quota for the day.

Antioxidants May Be Helpful

The latest research indicates that certain antioxidants (vitamins A, C, E, and beta carotene) may be beneficial. Antioxidants may protect us by protecting our cells or extending the life of the cells from oxidants produced by chemical reactions in the body.

Vitamin E may have a beneficial effect on the heart by preventing or reversing the deposits of cholesterol in the walls of the arteries (see p. 35).

Exercise

While exercise is not a dietary change, it is a necessary lifestyle change that you must make if you expect to notice any difference in your weight and your energy level. Studies show that exercise may increase your level of HDL—the "good"—cholesterol.

Chapter 6 discusses exercise for a healthy heart. Perform the exercise daily along with maintaining the low-fat, high-complex-carbohydrate eating plan for good health. You will notice a difference in the way you look and, most important, in the way you feel.

Table 7.11
Ways to Burn Calories with Activity

Activity	*Minutes to burn 100 calories*
bicycling	26 (6 mph.)
cleaning house	27
cooking meals	37
dancing	34 (slow)
dancing	12 (fast)
dusting	41
ironing	53
jogging	13 (5 mph.)
mowing lawn (power)	29
stationary cycling	16 (10 mph.)
swimming	30
typing	59
vacuuming	19
walking	27 (3 mph.)
walking	18 (4 mph.)
washing windows	29

IT'S UP TO YOU!

Starting and maintaining a low-fat, high-complex-carbohydrate weight control program may not be easy at first. Making plans to become more active, including starting the daily exercise program outlined in chapter 5, will be a difficult lifestyle change for some people. But studies show that those who stay on low-fat diets over six months gradually find that their tastes gravitate toward foods that are naturally low in fat. And people who begin exercising start to look forward to it after a few weeks.

This chapter has offered you some basic suggestions on how to begin eating for a healthy heart. Take these ideas and implement them in your daily routine today. As you plan your weekly menu, make low-fat, high-complex-carbohydrate choices. Most important, don't keep around your kitchen foods that will cause you to fail.

It's up to you! Winning with heart attack may involve some drastic lifestyle changes—changes only *you* can make. But the rewards of being able to lead an active, normal life without the worry of additional heart problems are well worth the sacrifice.

8

Coping with Stress

We don't want to hear this, but stress is here to stay. Whether it comes from demanding employers, screaming kids, or aggressive drivers during rush hour, stress can sneak up on us and sap all our energy. Most of the time we don't even realize we are stressed out . . . until we burn out, or, as in the case of 1.5 million Americans each year, until we have a heart attack.

Stress can show itself through a wide variety of physical changes and emotional responses, and these symptoms vary greatly from one person to the next. Perhaps the most universal sign of stress is a feeling of being pressured or overwhelmed.

RECOGNIZE THE WARNING SIGNS

Symptoms of stress vary greatly from one person to the next; aside from a feeling of being pressured or overwhelmed, symptoms may include:

- physical complaints: stomach aches, headaches, or diarrhea

- problems getting along with others

- changes in behavior: outbursts of temper, unexplained anger, crying for no reason, or withdrawal

- regression, behavior that is not age-appropriate

- disturbed sleep patterns: nightmares, too little or too much sleep

- impatience: you seem to have a short circuit in your behavior patterns.

If you are experiencing a number of these characteristics, chances are good that your level of stress is excessive. If left untreated, stress can lead to permanent feelings of helplessness and ineffectiveness.

HAVING SAFE STRESS

Researchers are defining the intricacies of the mind-body connection, as well as such effective "inner healing" methods as relaxation techniques, mental imagery or visualization, and attitude adjustment exercises. These methods can help keep stress in check so the body can function properly.

The main strategy in dealing with stress is to identify and remove or reduce its source. Identification may be relatively easy, but elimination could be a challenge, especially when the source of stress is your job. So it is important to find ways to reduce the level of stress. Relaxation, including deep breathing, muscle stretching and meditation, will help you practice safer stress.

DEEP BREATHING FOR RELAXATION

An acute or prolonged tense state may cause an increase in heart rate and blood pressure, dry mouth, enlarged pupils, sweaty palms, and fast, shallow "chest" breathing. However, slow, deep "abdominal" breathing helps break the tension cycle, which enables body functions to return to normal. Taking ten slow, deep breaths at tense times, as well as throughout the day, will help you to stay loose and relaxed (see Relaxation Response below).

Relaxation Response

Achieving relaxation through the relaxation response is important in helping to reduce some of the emotional stress of heart attack and daily living. The use of the relaxation response came from research showing that it can reduce stress, anxiety, tension, and pain developing a sense of inner quiet and peacefulness, a calming of negative thoughts and worries.

Relaxation response can be very helpful in heart attack, the experience of which, or even being at high risk and living in fear of a heart attack, is a major source of stress, both physically and mentally. Heart attack can affect one's mood, causing irritability, impatience, and higher levels of frustration. As will be discussed in this chapter, depression commonly occurs as well.

While heart attack is thought of as a physical problem, it is also known that fears and emotional factors can play a contributory role in the experience. For example, think of the people who accidentally cut a finger but do not experience pain until they look at their finger and are alarmed to see the blood! Fear in a heart attack can cause an increase in heart rate, which makes the heart do even more work!

Relaxation Can Be Learned

Relaxation can offer a real potential both for reducing physical strain and negative thoughts, and for increasing your ability to self-manage stress. Each of these capabilities has a positive effect on your heart.

Relaxation involves a mental approach to activity in general rather than any one specific activity. For each of us, many different activities or routines may be relaxing, depending on our particular mental attitude: what may relax one person can be frustrating or tension-producing for another. For example, some of us find it calming and soothing to lie quietly and listen to a certain type of music; others gain more relaxation from reading an enjoyable book. Remember that true relaxation involves more than simply lying still or engaging in some physical activity. You may not be relaxed simply by sitting in front of the TV. Some people even have a high level of tension in their bodies and minds during sleep. An example would be those who toss and turn at night or who grind their teeth during asleep.

Relaxation is a skill that everyone has the potential to develop. Some of us are naturally better at relaxing than others, but we can all learn to relax more effectively. Much like learning to play the piano or tennis, becoming good at relaxation takes time, patience, and practice. Learning to relax deeply and effectively is a skill that develops gradually and cannot be rushed or hurried.

Just Twenty Minutes a Day

To begin your own relaxation program, you might try the following steps. During some part of your day, set aside a period of about twenty minutes that you can devote to relaxation practice. This can be in the morning, afternoon or evening; just pick a time when you have few obligations or commitments so you won't feel hurried or rushed.

As much as possible, remove outside distractions that can disrupt your concentration: turn off the radio, the television, even the ringer on the telephone, if need be. During practice, it is important to either lie flat or recline comfortably so that your whole body is supported, relieving as much tension or tightness in your muscles as possible. Relieving tension is difficult to do while standing or sitting upright, since your muscles must be tightened to maintain the position. You can use a pillow or cushion under your head if this helps.

During the twenty-minute period, remain as still as possible; try to direct your thoughts away from the day's events. Focus your thoughts as much as you can on the immediate moment, and eliminate any outside thoughts that may compete for your attention. Try to focus entirely on yourself and the different kinds of feelings or sensations you may notice throughout your body. Take note of which parts of your body feel relaxed and loose, and which tense and tight.

Picture Your Body at Peace

As you go through these steps, try in your own way to imagine that every muscle in your body is now becoming loose, relaxed, and free of any excess tension. Picture all the muscles in your body beginning to unwind; imagine them going loose and limp.

As you do this, concentrate on making your breathing even, breathing slowly and regularly. With each breath you exhale, picture your muscles becoming even more relaxed, as if you were somehow breathing the tension away. At the end of twenty minutes, take a few moments to study and focus on the feelings and sensations you have been able to achieve. Notice whether areas that felt tight and tense at first now feel more loose and relaxed, and whether any areas of tension or tightness remain.

Don't be surprised if the relaxed feeling you achieved begins to fade and dissipate once you get up and return to your normal activities. Many people find that it is only after several weeks of daily, consistent practice that they can maintain the relaxed feeling beyond the practice session itself.

A variety of formal or structured approaches to relaxation training can be effective. One of these widely used techniques is progressive muscle relaxation, beginning with one area of the body and slowly moving to all other areas. Other methods are controlled breathing exercises, the use of mental imagery, and meditation (see below).

If you find it hard to relax on your own, or if you are interested in learning more about an individual approach for relaxation and stress management, it would be a good idea to see a clinical psychologist who specializes in these problems. Whether you use the techniques we have discussed or choose formal training by a professional, learning to relax effectively can help control the emotional stress of heart attack, increase positive thinking, and lessen the impact of this stress on your overall lifestyle.

MEDITATION*

A stress releaser called meditation is described as restful alertness; integration of mind, body and spirit; focused silence; and a form of prayer. It is not possible to clear the mind of negative beliefs or thoughts at a purely intellectual level. However, meditation is a powerful technique that guides you beyond the negative thoughts and agitations of the busy mind. It allows you to become "unstuck" from your fear and other disturbing emotions. The effectiveness of meditation was studied from a medical point of view by Herbert Benson, M.D., author of several wellness books. One of the studies involved the practice of Transcendental Meditation (TM) in patients with hypertension, a major risk factor for heart attack. These patients sat quietly for twenty minutes twice a day, before breakfast and dinner. They repeated a special word or mantra silently to themselves, allowing their thoughts to come and go. Dr. Benson observed a significant drop in their blood pressure from borderline high to normal range.

Other studies have shown that practicing meditation on a regular basis helps to relieve general fatigue and the stress that can lead to heart attacks and strokes.

VISUALIZATION

Another effective mind-body technique is mental imagery or visualization. Basically, this involves the power of your imagination using sights, sounds, feelings and smell to create a desired state in your mind.

---

*The information contained in this section is drawn from Patty Carroscia, R.N., *The Mind-Body Connection* (Jacksonville, Fla.: The Mind-Body Connection, 1992).

BALANCING YOUR LIFE:
ADVICE TO THE WORKAHOLIC

As you begin to think about the stress you are under and take steps to lessen this risk factor for heart attack, you must begin to balance your life. There is an old saying that no one on his deathbed ever wished he had spent more time at the office. Fortunately, you don't have to wait until then to realize that you may need to change your life.

Most of us can easily recognize the compulsive and addictive behavior of alcoholics, drug addicts, overeaters, and gamblers. We also recognize that these are serious problems requiring professional help. We may even acknowledge that other "normal" behaviors (TV watching, shopping, sex, cleanliness, or physical fitness) reflect internal problems requiring help when they are practiced in excess.

However, most people who work long hours would vehemently argue that they do so because of situational circumstances and necessity, not because they have a problem. They would deny that their behavior is compulsive or addictive and would claim that if they were to win the lottery tomorrow, they would readily demonstrate a different lifestyle.

It is important to note that workaholics are both men and women, employed outside or in the home, young and old. Yes, workaholics can be found in all walks of life. The homemaker who feels compelled about keeping a spotless house, cooking gourmet meals, baking her own bread, and ironing the sheets and underwear may be a workaholic when the action is addictive or compulsive, and interferes with the rest of her life and relationships.

The workaholic typically comes from a family where he or she enjoyed the role of the "good" kid and where being successful was valued and promoted. The fear of not being good enough or disappointing someone literally drives the workaholic to keep at it in order to hide deep-seated feelings of inadequacy and fear of "messing up."

Masked Feelings

On the surface, the workaholic often is viewed as successful, motivated, committed, and responsible. These outwardly positive signs are actually masking the underlying fears and insecurities.

Through hard work, the workaholic has found a method of altering painful and confusing feelings, including fears of failure, victimization, or losing control, among others.

The mood-altering experience of workaholism becomes so intense and captivating that it takes on a life of its own; it becomes difficult or impossible to control and dramatically affects others.

Dealing with Relationships

Predictably the workaholic usually develops problems in intimate relationships because things are functionally out of balance. Often the workaholic's spouse practices the same co-dependent behavior as the alcoholic (excuses and justifications made to explain canceled dinner parties, rationalizations of "he or she's just too tired to have sex," or "we need the money to get the kids through college.")

Frequent arguments, communication difficulties, or feelings of loneliness and isolation become identifiable problems in relationships. Essential to bringing about change is the understanding that working hard provides an emotional payoff to the workaholic and that the family system often supports the dysfunction.*

There Is Help

When working too long and too hard each day increases the stress in your life, you place yourself at greater risk for heart attack. Many heart attack victims fall into the category of the "workaholic." Now we realize there are still a lot of people who are hard workers and love what they do. Simply having some of the symptoms or reflecting some of the characteristics we have mentioned does not mean one is a workaholic. The healthy individual uses work to enhance life; the workaholic, on the other hand, uses work to survive (see the warning signs listed below). Often it takes someone other than yourself to see the difference.

Talk with your doctor about your work habits if you feel you have many of the warning signs of a workaholic. Using the Relaxation Response on pp. 146–49 and other tips for stress reduction, get your life back in balance.

Warning Signs of a Workaholic

- You love those twelve to fifteen hours a day at the office.

- You always have a briefcase full of papers to review.

---

*See Roger B. Szuch, L.C.S.W., *All Work and No Play . . . Is Your Life Out of Balance?* (Living Well Publications, Inc. 1992).

- You need to stay up after everyone has gone to bed to finish one more project.

- You haven't had a vacation in years and the last time you went, you couldn't wait to get home and return to work.

- You used to enjoy going to the beach with the family, boating, or dancing, but haven't had the time lately.

- You find Sundays difficult to endure.

- You can't relax.

- At home, your thoughts are on what needs to be done at the office.

- You feel pressured or angry about money.

- Your spouse and children don't really know you anymore and, for that matter, you don't know them very well, either.

- You haven't been truly intimate with your spouse in months.

- You are not feeling appreciated or understood.

- You may be eating and/or drinking too much.

- You promise to slow down, but never do.

REGAINING CONTROL OF YOUR LIFE

It is frightening to be at a high risk for heart attack, and even more frightening to have experienced a heart attack and to worry incessantly about it happening again. You may have expressed to loved ones or to your physician that "living with heart attack (or fear of one) is like no life at all." Your problems are very real, and they often have a devastating effect on your outlook on life and your daily activities.

We have given you some of the negative areas you might experience with heart attack. By reviewing each of these negative areas you can develop very effective strategies for coping with them for better enjoyment of life.

Please read each topic with an open mind. There are ways in which you *can* have an impact on your life. There are areas you *can* change, as well as definite alternatives to reliance only on medical intervention.

Acceptance

As a heart attack patient or as someone with high risk factors for heart attack, your ultimate goal is to reach the point where you can accept this reality, and then make modifications to handle it within your life.

The opposite of acceptance is *denial.* Denial is the behavior that works against heart attack rehabilitation effort. An illustrative example of this is the heart attack patient who tried to conduct business as usual from his room in the coronary care unit! It is vital to your rehabilitation that you accept the fact that nonmedical issues such as suspicion, anxiety, anger, or loss of self-esteem can and do affect your life and level of stress you encounter each day. If you are not willing to admit this, you will have no reason to engage in any type of rehabilitation therapy.

Denial or nonacceptance is often an attempt to preserve self-esteem. You may think that if you admit that something other than a physical problem is increasing stress, your friends and family will think that it is psychological or something you have fabricated. This is certainly not the case. Stress factors in the family or even at work can affect all areas of your life—your thoughts, your outlook, and, yes, even your perception of wellness after a heart attack. Acceptance is the first step in successful rehabilitation.

Survival Strategies for Reaching Acceptance

1. *Keep an open mind on nonmedical treatment.* A variety of treatments, such as relaxation and biofeedback, are available and can easily be learned. We have already mentioned meditation, visualization, and the relaxation response in this chapter. These stress managers really do work! See the relaxation response information on pp. 146–49 and practice it daily until you are able to use this tool whenever you feel anxious.

2. *Do not feel that, because you are seeing a counselor, your friends or family members will think the stress of heart attack is something you imagined.* Psychological intervention can often bring relief from the stress of heart disease when medical treatment has failed. How you react to stressors in your life can be helped by a qualified therapist as you learn positive coping skills.

3. *Keep a daily record of your feelings and the intensity of your stress.* Ask a counselor or your doctor to look at this diary and help you work through the overwhelming moments by changing negative behaviors or actions.

4. *Accept your stress.* This does not mean that you have to "like" the stress you are experiencing, but acceptance will allow you to redirect your life as you begin to manage it in an appropriate manner. As you begin coping techniques and the medical treatment plan as directed by your physician, you will experience reduced stress, which will be an unanticipated benefit.

Coping with Constant Anxiety and Fears

Every heart attack patient or person at risk for heart attack can experience feelings of anxiety and fear. The fears can be very real, and usually involve questions about the future:

- Will my chances of heart attack worsen?

- Can I handle the increased stress of living with this condition?

- Will I become homebound?

- Will my friends leave me alone with my suffering?

- Will I be able to keep my job?

- How can I wake up each day with the fears I have?

- Will I be able to care for my family if I have a heart attack?

Becoming obsessive about your fears—dwelling on what *may* happen—will make it difficult to move in a positive direction. It is far better to recognize your fears and redirect your energy toward optimistic behaviors in order to stop or change the negative thoughts and actions. Worrying about what cannot be changed will only make you more anxious and fearful.

Survival Strategies for Ending Anxiety and the Fear of Heart Attack

1. *Write down those situations that make you anxious and fearful.* These may include a certain program or newscast on television, a friend who is negative, conflict with a family member who does not accept your condition, or even reading the morning paper. Try to avoid these encounters whenever possible, so that you are not confronted with fear or stress.

2. *Do not expect your family or friends to be your therapists.* Find a licensed mental health counselor and make an appointment to "talk it out" with an impartial trained professional who understands these problems.

3. *Keep an open mind about legitimate nonmedical interventions that can help you relax.* These may include as biofeedback, relaxation response, music therapy, and others.

4. *Join a support group of heart attack patients.* If there is no support group in your area, talk with your physician about starting one. Take the initiative to help yourself.

5. *Ask your physician to explain the nature of heart disease to your family, including why there are some days you do better than other days.* This will help your family to become more understanding and empathic when your level of stress and anxiety or even the pain of angina is high.

Coping with Suspicion

Living positively with heart attack can make you more sensitive to the thoughts and actions of others. Constant, unrelenting fear day after day may result in distorted thoughts and behavior. This does not mean that you are crazy, but that the stress has affected the way you interpret what people do and say.

If you find yourself becoming overly suspicious, sit back and consider the possibility that you are overreacting to a person or situation. Ask a trusted friend or counselor about your accusations, but be sure you are going to listen to the response and not berate your listener for having a different opinion.

We are not asking you to be naive about people and their motives. Instead, we want you to realize that living with heart attack or with the fear of having heart attack is often stressful enough to distort your thinking.

Survival Strategies for Suspicion

1. Relearn to trust others.

2. Even if people are doing and saying things you do not like, do not let it bother you to the point of not accepting their word.

3. Confront others with your suspicions. If they have a reasonable response, believe them.

4. Remember that harboring negative thoughts about others (even if such thoughts are true) is detrimental to your health and general outlook on life.

5. Look carefully at those people who arouse your suspicion, and see whether there is an alterative explanation for their actions.

Coping with Anger and Irritability

While anger is a natural reaction to heart attack or the fear associated with heart disease, ways of coping with the anger can vary from one person to another. Some use the anger in a positive manner, some ignore it, and others let angry feelings consume them. In order to cope with the anger and irritability that often accompanies heart attack, it will help you to try and understand these feelings better. Once you do, you can replace the energy you spend being angry with positive actions to make life more enjoyable both for yourself and for those around you.

If you have lived with the nagging fear of heart attack for months or years, you definitely have a right to be angry, but you do not have the right to hurt others while expressing this anger.

Survival Strategies for Anger and Irritability

1. Anger, if not expressed in a positive manner, is an emotion that can destroy your health. It is important to realize that anger can injure your body.

2. Anger is an emotion that everyone is entitled to feel at times, but again, it is important to express this in a way that will neither be detrimental to your overall health and well-being nor hurt those around you.

3. If anger is consuming your entire day, realize that you need to find some ways of changing this.

4. Even if your anger does get out of control on a "bad" day, stop immediately and apologize to those around you.

5. Write down those situations or persons who create angry feelings in you. Try to avoid getting into these situations if you feel you might explode.

6. Ask your physician to recommend a professional who can give you some tools for coping with angry feelings.

Coping with Loss of Control

In addition to feelings of anger and irritability, heart attack can cause loss of control over many other aspects of your life that once depended on your abilities, ideas, or strength, but no longer do. Instead of being in charge of your own destiny, you may feel as if heart attack has control of you, as though you were a puppet on a string.

There is a fine line between what you *think* you cannot control and what you absolutely cannot control. The key to dealing effectively with this problem is to make sure you understand where these two areas differ. The following survival strategies offer some solutions.

Survival Strategies for Loss of Control

1. *Make a list of factors you want to change in your life.* With the help of your physician, mental health counselor, family and friends, start applying yourself to those areas in your life that you still have control over.

2. *If something, such as work, becomes too much to handle and you must give it up, do not get stressed over this situation.* Talk to someone about your feelings and fears, and learn to channel these feelings into another direction that you *do* have control over.

3. *If you need help with an area that you have lost control over, such as housecleaning or driving to the doctor, ask for help.* It is not a sign of personal failure to obtain assistance from someone—we all need help at some time in our lives.

4. *Set goals each day to tackle a new area that you can control.* Perhaps you have been unable to begin an exercise program due to unfounded fears that this may put you at greater risk of heart attack. If your doctor agrees, start by deciding to walk one block at a time and try to tackle this task. As you walk the block successfully, take your pulse. Is your breathing and heart rate regular and within normal range of exertion? Gradually increase your walking as your doctor suggests.

Soon you may be able to regain control over exercise as a method of treatment and prevention of heart attack. You can approach other areas in your life in the same way—one step at a time—until you can begin to *live the life you deserve*. Remember, taking one small step at a time will let you regain control and confidence over those areas that have been beyond reach for some time.

Coping with Avoidance Behaviors

From the time we are infants, we learn to avoid painful actions. If we touched a hot grill and were burned, we learned to stay clear of hot grills. It is a natural reaction to avoid pain. Until recently, it was the right thing to do.

Now that you have had a heart attack or suffer fears of having one, the whole scenario changes. If you constantly avoid stress or activity, you will become inactive. When you are inactive, you increase your chances of not getting well—remember, heart muscles must be exercised to function properly. Does this sound like a vicious circle to you? It is!

You *must* allow yourself to move, exercise, and face the normal stresses of daily living in order to get better. All these avoidance behaviors are not helping, at least not in the long run. In behaving this way, you only get short-term relief for a long-term problem.

Survival Strategies for Reducing Avoidance Behaviors

1. Make yourself perform at least one activity a day that you would have avoided in the past.

2. Force yourself to participate in one leisure activity a week with family or friends.

3. Never ask anyone else to do for you what you are capable of doing for yourself.

Coping with Social Isolation

Social isolation may be a three-faceted problem for you. First of all, you are purposely avoiding some people due to fatigue, irritability, or the many other problems you have to face each day with heart attack. You find your home a secure haven where you are not on display and where there are loved ones around to meet your needs.

Second, there may be friends who are purposely avoiding you. It is possible that you have driven them away by continually focusing upon your physical problems. They may be kind and ask about your health, but long lectures on the latest surgery or treatments are not what friends willingly want to hear over and over again.

Third, for some people, leaving the bed or house can be associated with wellness. As we explained earlier, you may be fearful that some people who see you "out and about" may assume you are back to "normal." Once you are considered better, family and friends may be quick to expect you to do things you are incapable of doing.

Survival Strategies for Social Isolation

1. Look out for nonverbal cues or body language that suggest people are tuning you out as you talk about your heart attack or fears.

2. Limit these "me-related" conversations to five minutes.

3. Never turn you back on true friends—they are an important support system.

4. When people ask "How are you feeling today?" do not mistake this for an interest in hearing all the details of how bad you feel.

5. Make yourself go on at least one outing each weekend and one during the week—more if possible, but at least one a week.

Coping with Self-Centered Orientation

When someone goes into the hospital for heart surgery or diagnostic testing, family members focus on helping until the patient is up and about again. However, even after the problem has become chronic and gone on for months or years, some patients continue to expect everyone's life to revolve around theirs, and some families continue to provide this service. It is difficult to change such a pattern once it becomes routine. While you never intended to be a burden on anyone, you may have fallen into a pattern of focusing solely on yourself. It is easy to do so when all thoughts and actions revolve around you.

If this routine has occurred in your home, do not place blame on either side. Instead, talk with your family and begin to initiate changes that are more family-oriented than self-centered.

Coping Strategies for Changing a Self-Centered Orientation

1. Eliminate certain statements from your interactions with others, including:

(a) "My problems are the worst."

(b) "No one knows how I feel."

(c) "If this ever happens to you, you'll be sorry for how you've treated me."

2. Take time each day to focus on the problem of someone else in your family; do not allow yourself to be the constant center of attention.

3. In social situations, try to eliminate all reference to your heart problem or past heart attack.

4. If there is a difference of opinion as to whether or not you have become self-centered, consider family therapy to iron out the variance in viewpoints.

Coping with Communication Problems

How is it that your family says you never hear what they say, or hear it incorrectly? Being fearful due to heart disease can easily take your mind off the subject of conversation. You may actually have gotten into the habit of not listening, thinking that whatever was said will come up again later.

Moreover, you may be experiencing memory problems due to lack of attention and concentration or poor sleep. Though you may be experiencing some or all of these problems, it is very important that you work to keep open and clear lines of communication with your family and loved ones. If they feel that you are not listening to them (for whatever reasons), they will be less inclined to listen to you.

Survival Strategies for Communication Problems

1. *Listen* to others when they talk.

2. Ask questions if you are not clear about the details of what is being said.

3. Be direct. Do not assume, for example, that others will automatically know that you do not want company on the weekend.

4. Avoid indirect communication or body language such as grimaces, slamming doors, sarcasm, or pouting.

5. Consider a community education course on "Enhancing Communication Skills." (Check with your local community health center for dates and times.)

6. Consider family and/or marital counseling to help improve the communication system at home.

Coping with Abuse to the Family

You know that your family is most important to you, but it seems that you treat them worse than you would outsiders. Why is that? Through the years you have always been able to "let your hair down" at home. When you felt bad, it was acceptable to let your family members know since they would understand and make allowances for you. However, even now that you have experienced heart attack, it is not appropriate to continue to take things out on your loved ones day after day.

Survival Strategies for Abuse to Family

1. Try putting your family above outsiders and yourself.

2. On one day, pretend your family members are guests and treat them as such.

3. Monitor your angry responses and try to redirect your anger into creative outlets such as writing, playing an instrument, painting, cooking, or exercise.

4. Apologies are greatly appreciated. Do not assume that your family will know you are feeling remorseful.

5. Do not drive you family away. Remember, when the chips are down, they are the ones who will always be there.

Coping with Stress

"Stressed out" is a term used to describe the impact that life stressors have on you. These stressors include anxiety, tension, high blood pressure, depression, and anger—all increasing your risk for heart attack. As a heart patient, you experience stressors across all aspects of your life: physical stressors (the pain), social stressors (loss of friends and activities), work stressors (loss of job or difficulty working), and family stressors (feelings of dependency on others).

You have every right to be stressed, but this does not mean that you cannot do anything about it.

Survival Strategies for Decreasing Stress

1. Write down the very things that make you "stressed," including situations, people, and others. Make a conscious effort to avoid those areas you have no control over.

2. If you are experiencing any physical symptoms of stress, such as high blood pressure, headaches, or anxiety attacks, be sure to consult your physician. See chapter 5 for ways to reduce hypertension, and stay on the medication your physician prescribes.

3. Take a class on stress management offered through your community center or a local wellness program.

4. A therapist who specializes in stress management can help teach you ways of dealing with overwhelming problems, people, and situations.

5. Try using relaxation tapes, which are available at local book stores, or learn how to do the relaxation response outlined on pp. 146–49. Use this type of therapy when you feel your body becoming tense.

Coping with Depression

Depression is very debilitating: it ruins the lives of thousands of people after heart attack. Perhaps you don't feel depressed, but this does not mean you're not experiencing depression. Depressive symptoms can include:

- disturbed in sleep patterns
- loss of interest in usual activities
- weight loss or gain (more than 5 percent of body weight)
- fatigue
- thoughts of dying or suicide
- irritability
- mood swings
- staying at home all the time

- avoiding special friends

- reduced or increased appetite

- difficulty concentrating

Some people with heart attack, however, may be well aware that they are depressed; they experience uncontrollable tearfulness, feelings of helplessness and/or hopelessness, loss of self-worth, and suicidal thoughts or plans. If you have these feelings, you must contact a professional to get help.

Survival Strategies for Combating Depression

1. See a qualified mental health specialist if you feel you are being immobilized by depression.

2. If you have suicidal thoughts, talk them out with someone. Never keep these thoughts to yourself.

3. Use only medication prescribed by your physician. Alcohol and illicit drugs cannot combat depression.

4. Since exercise can help to ease depression, determine what you can do physically and begin to get active. Talk with your doctor about the exercise program described in this book, and see if you can begin this treatment for depression.

5. Stick to a fixed routine each day. Staying in bed all day, unless advised by your doctor, cannot help you alleviate the depressive feelings.

Coping with Loss of Self-Esteem

Sometimes heart attack can affect the pride you have in yourself. It often leads to job loss, decreased contact with friends, and reduction in leisure pursuits. For many of us, our entire self-esteem is wrapped up in one or all of these activities. Now, when someone asks, "What do you do?" you may not respond with: "I'm a sales manager," or "I am an attorney," or "I am a teacher." Instead, you may think to yourself, "I am a failure" or "I sit home all day." When you no longer have an occupation with which to identify, your self-worth may suffer.

Being with friends and doing things for them and your family may have been your whole identity. Instead of being able to take an entire meal over to a sick friend or driving your neighbor to have his car fixed, you are the one who needs help. If you have been a very in-dependent individual, this switch to dependency has probably taken its toll on your self-esteem.

Survival Strategies for Combating Low Self-Esteem

1. Take your focus off the negative aspects of your life.

2. Make a list of all your good qualities.

3. Remember that your family loves you for more than the paycheck you brought home.

4. Allow yourself to consider less demanding jobs that would occupy your time and make you feel worthwhile.

5. Do not avoid social interactions. In the end this only isolates you and makes you feel worse.

6. Try to do as many things for yourself as you can. You will feel better the more independent you become.

Coping with Physical Ailments

We all know that when we feel bad, our outlook on life takes on a negative perspective, and petty issues appear to be insurmountable problems. Although you most likely had some physical ailments before your heart attack, you were emotionally capable of handling them. This may be the first major long-term or life-threatening illness you have had to deal with.

Additional problems associated with your heart attack can create other physical ailments. For example, hypertension is the leading risk factor for heart attack; it is also a known risk factor in stroke and kidney disease. Uncontrolled diabetes, another a risk factor in heart attack, can also lead to blindness, loss of limbs, and kidney failure.

Survival Strategies for Avoiding Other Physical Ailments

1. Go to a physician about additional problems to help ease your mind. If he says it is not serious, believe him.

2. Consider nonmedical alternatives such as relaxation techniques, counseling, and biofeedback.

3. Avoid "doctor shopping."

4. Consider a physician-approved exercise program so that your body can begin getting well, thereby reducing your risk factors for future problems.

YOU *CAN* WIN!

You may have experienced several of the stressful issues we have described in this chapter, and some may seem insurmountable. This is not so! You can maintain or regain control of your life and *win* with heart attack. You can make changes in both your thinking and your behavior. Do not feel that you must do this alone. There are trained professionals ready to guide you and your family in a positive direction. Ask for help—you will be glad you did.

9

From Patient to Person

Every day there are people winning against heart attack. Many realize that they can help prevent the most common cause of death in America by taking simple preventive measures. Others, who have suffered from heart attack and angina pectoris, have taken steps to lower their chance of future heart attack and death.

By checking your risk factors, taking steps to correct or limit each risk factor and following your doctor's advice, you can take control and begin to win. You can use the new facts and information about steps that work. Whether it's prevention of heart attack altogether or of another attack, you can make a difference in the outcome!

The following are true case studies of patients who are taking control, getting their lives back and winning against heart attack.

UNSTABLE ANGINA

Fred R. is a 49-year-old salesman. He became worried when he noticed discomfort in his chest that lasted a few minutes at a time when he walked up a flight of stairs. He ignored the feeling for a few weeks, but after the pain started when he was walking to his car, he became worried enough to ask for a medical opinion.

Fred was fifty pounds overweight, his blood pressure was 175/100; and his blood cholesterol was 305, with LDL cholesterol of 200 and HDL cholesterol of 40. He had cut back on cigarettes to only a few per day over the last month because of worry over his condition.

An exercise electrocardiogram (ECG) was done which showed that Fred was experiencing chest discomfort along with abnormal changes on ECG, suggesting heart problems. A coronary arteriogram found a major blockage of the left anterior descending coronary artery. Fol-

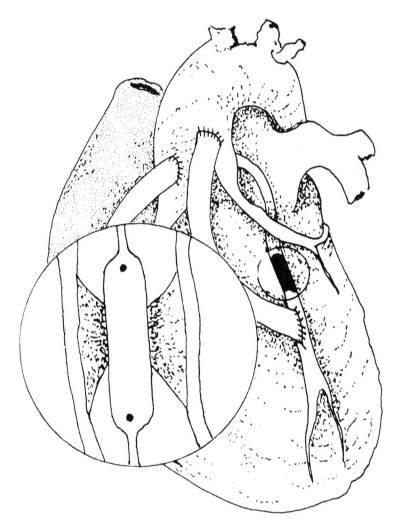

Figure 9.1
Balloon Angioplasty: As the balloon is expanded,
the blockage of the artery is reduced.

lowing balloon angioplasty (see figure 9.1) Fred has not experienced any chest discomfort.

After these treatments, Fred made some changes in his life. He has lost most of those fifty extra pounds, he takes medication to control his blood pressure and cholesterol, and hopes to be able to eliminate some of the medication with continued diet and weight loss.

Fred also began a walking exercise program, which has helped reduce weight. He tells of feeling better than he has in years. He takes one aspirin and a vitamin E supplement daily.

Fred's risk of heart attack was about twenty times higher than normal when he started treatment. By giving up cigarettes, and controlling hypertension and cholesterol, he dramatically reduced his future risk. Studies show that adding low doses of aspirin, as discussed on p. 112, and vitamin E supplements can lower the risk of heart attack. Fred was fortunate in that he sought treatment before a major heart attack caused permanent limitation or even death. His future now looks a lot brighter.

ACUTE MYOCARDIAL INFARCTION

Sarah M., sixty-one, works as a secretary and has always enjoyed excellent health. She is not overweight and her blood pressure is usually around 130/80. Although Sarah's father died of a heart attack at age fifty-four, she had no other known risk factors for heart attack.

Sarah was admitted to a coronary care unit after she felt severe heaviness in her chest for two hours, with shortness of breath and sweating. She was found to have heart attack (acute myocardial infarction) but no other complications.

Sarah's cholesterol had not been checked in years. Her total cholesterol was found to be 289, with LDL cholesterol of 220 and HDL cholesterol of 40. She began a low cholesterol diet, and after two months her LDL cholesterol decreased to 180. She planned to continue her diet and add medication for cholesterol later if needed. Sarah took one aspirin and vitamin E supplements each day and began a daily exercise program with an exercise bicycle in her home. She also added estrogen supplements on the advice of her gynecologist.

Sarah's risk factors included a family history of heart attack and cholesterol levels which alone put her at more than double the risk of heart attack. Her LDL cholesterol was well above the recommended level of 130, while the HDL of 40 was lower than the desirable level of 60.

As we've said, around the time of menopause, the rate of heart attack increases in women. By age sixty-five, it catches up with the rate in men, in part due to the loss of estrogen at menopause, thus allowing a decrease in protection from HDL cholesterol. Also, LDL cholesterol tends to rise during these years, which also increases the heart risk.

Sarah made major changes in her risk status by controlling cholesterol, and adding estrogen and exercise as well as aspirin and vitamin E. As discussed in chapters 2 and 5, each of these steps clearly lowers the risk of heart attack, some by 40 percent or more!

EXCESS WEIGHT AND EXERCISE

Jamal V., forty-six, had been overweight most of his life. Two years ago his father died suddenly of a heart attack at age sixty-five while playing golf. Looking at his own risk factors, Jamal realized that his eighty-five pounds of excess weight put him at higher heart risk also. His blood pressure was 130/78 and his cholesterol tests showed total cholesterol of 250, LDL cholesterol of 155, HDL cholesterol of 35, and triglycerides at 485.

Jamal decided to start dieting to lose weight; but after three months, he had lost only two pounds. Then he read that exercise can help with weight loss, so he began walking. Jamal started with one or two blocks, and after a few weeks was walking over a mile each day. After a few months of diet and walking, he had lost fourteen pounds.

Over the next six months Jamal lost another thirty-five pounds; he found his energy improved and felt much more productive in his work as an accountant. His triglycerides on repeat testing dropped to 210, his LDL cholesterol was 133, and his HDL cholesterol increased to 50.

Jamal's risk factors were excess weight, family history of heart disease, high triglycerides, high LDL cholesterol and low HDL cholesterol in addition to lack of regular exercise. His self-determination actually got him started on the path to much lower risk for heart attack and death.

Excess weight, as discussed on pp. 40–41, increases the risk of heart disease, and often brings with it high triglycerides and cholesterol. For Jamal, his inactive lifestyle was creating major problems. Diet alone wasn't successful; but when he added a simple walking program the weight loss began because Jamal was using up or "spending" more calories than he was taking in each day.

As a result of exercise and weight control, Jamal's triglycerides and LDL cholesterol fell as expected. HDL cholesterol increased—some studies show that walking even eight to ten miles per week can help raise HDL cholesterol.

Jamal took steps to take charge of his health, including his risk of heart attack and death. As extra benefits, he felt more energetic and was more productive at work.

STRESS AND HIGH BLOOD PRESSURE

Rodney J. is a 47-year-old vice president of a large manufacturing corporation. During a routine physical exam he found that his blood pressure was 150/94. Since Fred was nervous during the exam, which found no other abnormalities, his doctor suggested he take his blood pressure at home. Several readings with a blood pressure cuff at home over the next two weeks showed the same level or higher.

Rodney was under stress at work, traveled most days of the week, and had concerns about his job security. His mother, who lived in a city a thousand miles away, was ill, and his job situation put pressure on his marriage. Rodney, who always drank several cups of coffee each day, had increased his intake recently. Minor stresses now seemed to cause much more worry and nervousness than they once had. Rodney had trouble sleeping, was more impatient with his children, and always felt tired.

Rodney probably was suffering from the effects of stress, which actually caused his blood pressure to rise. Many of his feelings were likely due to stress, including irritability, nervousness, insomnia, impatience, and fatigue. Studies show that damage to blood vessels may gradually increase as the blood pressure rises above 120/80. In any case, it is clear that with blood pressure above 140/90 the risk of heart disease and other cardiovascular disease at least doubles.

While many of life's daily stresses can't be stopped, we can control *how we respond* to the stress. As in Rodney's case, stress can actually raise blood pressure, thereby increasing the risks of heart attack and death!

Rodney discussed his situation with a clinical psychologist who specializes in stress management. He was given some suggestions about how to cope and manage his stress, and learned to practice the *relaxation response* (see pp. 146–49). In twenty-minute sessions each day, Rodney was able to greatly reduce his feelings of stress. He even practiced the relaxation response on the plane as he traveled.

After reviewing and controlling his other risk factors, Rodney also began a regular exercise program. Since then he feels much more in control of his life: His blood pressure has decreased to its former level of 125/82, and it is likely that Rodney's stress management as well as his other steps have controlled his blood pressure. With his pressure now in control, Rodney has greatly improved his future health outlook.

TYPE A PERSONALITY

Robert B., a hard-driving owner of a chain of fast food restaurants, recently had his routine health checkup. Although he had no new major problems identified, he continued to appear stressed most of the time. Robert completed a short questionnaire listing factors noticed in "type A" personalities. He answered affirmatively to most of the questions noted below.

- Are you hard-driving and competitive?

- Do you usually feel pressed for time?

- Do other people consider you bossy and dominating?

- Do you feel a strong need to excel in most things?

- Do you eat quickly?

- Do you often think about work after hours?

- Do you often feel your work stretches you to your limits of energy and capacity?

- Do you often feel uncertain or dissatisfied with how well you're doing?

- Do you get upset when you have to wait for something?

Affirmative responses to these questions identify those classified as "type A" personalities. The hurried, overachieving, hard-driving businessperson is a common example. Their risk of heart attack is higher, but just being busy and aggressive does not in itself bring a higher heart risk.

The specific problems of *hostility* and *anger* are those that increase the heart risk. Studies show that these feelings and actions can be changed if the problems are realized. Some simple techniques can actually lower hostility and anger! By recognizing and removing these risk factors, you can actually lower your own risk of heart attack.

If your answer is "yes" to most of the above questions, reread p. 110, assess your risk, and consider talking to a clinical psychologist to begin some simple steps to make a change. These are easy but important ways to control your future health and gain peace of mind.

BIRTH CONTROL PILLS AND SMOKING

Suzanne W. is a 39-year-old banking executive who smokes half a pack of cigarettes daily; she has also been taking birth control pills for the past ten years. She is not overweight, does not exercise regularly, and has normal blood pressure and normal cholesterol. Since her father had a heart attack at the age of sixty-five, Suzanne wondered about her own risk.

Suzanne's risk factors include family history of heart attack, smoking cigarettes, and taking birth control pills. With her father's history of heart attack, it would be a good idea for her to be careful about her other risk factors.

Smoking increases the risk of heart attack in women and men. Even "light" smoking—one to four cigarettes per day—increases the risk. And nonsmokers exposed to smoke have an even higher risk!

Of special concern in Suzanne's case is the combination of birth control pills and cigarettes. Some studies show up to 23 times the risk of heart attack in women who smoke *and* take contraceptives. Many of the newer combinations of birth control pills are less risky, but women should still be aware of this higher risk.

A regular exercise program would be a good idea for heart risk as well as for general well-being in Suzanne's case. A few steps now could prevent Suzanne from becoming a cardiac patient later.

STABLE ANGINA

Joseph M. is a 75-year-old retired schoolteacher. For five years he had had the sensation of tightness and heaviness under the breastbone when he hurried or walked uphill, but it went away when he rested or took nitroglycerin. When Joseph was first diagnosed with angina pectoris, he was worried about heart attack and limited his activity severely: He no longer went to visit his grandchildren or enjoyed other activities because of fear of bringing on a heart attack.

Then, as he learned more about his problem, Joseph found that he had more control than he originally thought. Looking at his risk factors, Joseph found that his blood pressure was 165/85, his cholesterol was 245 with LDL of 160 and HDL of 40, and he was about twenty pounds overweight.

After talking with his doctor, Joseph began medication for hypertension; his blood pressure dropped to 140/82. He made some adjustments in his diet to lower saturated fats and increase his olive oil consumption. He began taking one aspirin every other day, and he later even added a walking program. Joseph has improved over the past two years and is now enjoying his family, becoming much more active, and walking one to two miles each day. He rarely experiences chest discomfort now, even with more activity.

Joseph had stable angina pectoris but allowed it to severely limit his life. He found that he could improve his condition by looking at specific parts of the problem. He had systolic hypertension and began treatment. (In this form of hypertension the systolic [upper] number is above 160 while the diastolic [lower] number remains normal (see p. 20): This form of hypertension has been shown to be important as a risk factor for future heart disease.

Low doses of aspirin have been found to decrease the chance of second heart attack (see p. 112). This low dose does not usually cause side effects.

An exercise program is an important part of the treatment of coronary heart disease. It can even be begun in a cardiac rehabilitation program where heart monitors can make sure no problems go undetected. In the long run, Joseph will have a healthier heart; he has already lowered his risk of heart attack and death by his actions.

AUTOMATIC DEFIBRILLATOR

Scott P., who had already suffered two heart attacks, was following his doctor's advice, but he still had irregular heart beats at times. Medications were tried with some success. One day Scott suffered sudden cardiac arrest; fortunately some bystanders knew how to perform cardiopulmonary resuscitation (CPR) methods and kept his heart pumping until emergency medical services arrived.

In the hospital Scott had several episodes of dangerously irregular heatbeat. He eventually had a device implanted with electrodes connected to the heart. The device, called an Automatic Implanted Cardiac Defibrillator (AICD), automatically corrects the irregular heartbeat. Since then Scott has resumed all his usual daily activities, including travel. In the past year he has had two "firings" of his AICD when it detected an irregular heartbeat.

This device has allowed Scott to resume an almost normal life. He continues his doctor's advice to control the coronary heart disease and does everything possible to "prevent the next heart attack."

COLLAPSE

Skip M. was forty-eight when he found out about heart disease. At that time, Skip smoked one and a half packs of cigarettes daily, was about twenty pounds overweight, and hadn't checked his blood pressure or cholesterol in years. He was playing softball when he collapsed on the way to the dugout after scoring a run. With quick action by his teammates and the local rescue squad, Skip's condition was stabilized and later he was admitted to a coronary care unit with a heart attack.

Skip was fortunate. He survived his heart attack, even though there is an almost 50 percent chance of death in heart attacks before reaching the hospital. He began cardiac rehabilitation even before being discharged. Since then Skip has continued a regular exercise program, lost his excess weight, stopped smoking, started taking vitamin E and one aspirin per day, and has thereby greatly decreased his chances of a second heart attack. He found out his cholesterol was abnormal (total cholesterol 265, LDL of 188, and HDL of 34) and follows a diet with medications for cholesterol.

Men in their late forties are at risk for heart disease. Check your risk factors. With a few easy steps you may be able to prevent permanent damage, physical limitations, and death.

SUDDEN DEATH

Perry B. was a healthy, active man when at age forty-nine he collapsed and died on a running course near his home. The cause of death was found to be heart attack.

Is there any way to prevent this tragedy? Studies show that in a large percentage of cases such as this, there may be some warning signs, such as chest discomfort, which are ignored or overlooked. Although sudden death can occur in an otherwise healthy man with no risk factors, it is very uncommon. When examined closely, most of these cases show hypertension, abnormal cholesterol, smoking, or some combination of these risk factors.

In up to one-third of all cases, heart attack is the first sign of heart disease. If you don't check your own risk factors now, you may miss a great opportunity to prevent heart attack and possibly sudden death. No one wants to look for trouble, but in this case ignoring your own heart facts is like sticking your head in the sand.

PERSEVERANCE

Jane A., sixty-four years old, who has remained active despite some arthritis in her back and hips, began noticing an occasional burning sensation, like heartburn, in the left side of her chest, although it lasted only a few minutes. Jane had an upper gastrointestinal X-ray to look for stomach ulcer.

Jane continued to have the discomfort; when it became more frequent after walking or working, she began to limit her activity. She then had an exercise test which was normal. Because she noticed no improvement, Jane eventually underwent coronary angiography (discussed on p. 67). Jane was shown to have a major blockage in two coronary arteries. Following treatment she no longer had discomfort, and resumed her usual activities, including travel.

Jane's perseverance was justified; once the answer was found, her coronary heart disease was treated. It is common for symptoms to be confusing, so if you don't feel comfortable with the answer you're given, seek another doctor's opinion.

Studies show that over recent years some cardiac testing has been less common in women. This may be a result of the belief that coronary heart disease is less common in women than in men. However, at least 250,000 women die each year of coronary heart disease.

Chest discomfort or other unexplained symptoms should be evaluated equally in women and men until coronary heart disease and other serious problems have been ruled out.

SYNCOPE

Yvonne W. was sixty-six when she noticed dizziness which came on suddenly, but lasted only a few seconds. Then while doing yardwork, she fainted and seemed to lose consciousness for a brief time. Yvonne was then admitted to the hospital, where her heart was monitored. She was found to have periods of irregular heart beat caused by major blockage of a coronary artery (the left anterior descending).

Yvonne underwent coronary artery angioplasty; now, six years later, she suffers no further dizziness or blackouts. Her activity is not limited.

Yvonne experienced one of the well-known but less common manifestations of coronary heart disease. By monitoring her heartbeat, doctors were able to diagnose and treat Yvonne's condition. Through prompt action a potentially life-threatening problem was alleviated.

EXERCISE

Tony O. was fifty-four when he first found out that he had heart disease. He had a sedentary but stressful job driving a taxi for almost twenty years, was a little overweight, and smoked a pack of cigarettes daily. After the first snowstorm of the year, Tony was hurrying to shovel snow from his driveway to get his car out for work when he felt heaviness in his chest. He also felt short of breath and sweaty. He almost ignored these feelings, but decided to check with his doctor. Tony was found to have coronary heart disease with a major blockage of one coronary artery. He underwent successful angioplasty and within a short time was back driving his cab.

Tony started a regular exercise program and with great effort quit smoking cigarettes to help his heart. Since his work schedule changed often, he walked outside when he could and bought a treadmill for those times when he couldn't walk outside due to work or bad weather. Tony now walks about five miles a day and has lost over ten pounds.

The benefits of exercise are so great that a person in Tony's situation cannot ignore it any more than he can a prescribed medication. Regular exercise to increase fitness works! Some studies show that men who had higher level of fitness also had up to three times fewer deaths from coronary heart disease.

Exercise offers multiple benefits:

1. It can increase the HDL cholesterol as well as lower the LDL cholesterol, which lowers heart risk.

2. It helps lower blood pressure. In some cases of hypertension, a regular exercise program may even lower the blood pressure to such an extent that medication will not be needed.

3. It can help control excess weight. Exercising for just twenty minutes, three times each week can help reduce the amount of fat in the body. This would be about the amount of exercise in briskly walking three miles, or two to three miles of swimming or the equivalent amount of exercise. With exercise, your body will tend to lower more "fat" weight than "muscle" weight.

Start slowly, but check with your doctor first to be sure your plans are safe. Join a cardiac rehabilitation program if you already have heart disease. First, do only a few minutes of exercise, so you don't feel any worse when you finish than when you started. Then gradually increase as you can.

The long-term goal should be to walk ten to fifteen miles per week, to do thirty to fifty miles per week on a bicycle or exercise bike, or perform equivalent exercise. Other activities such as golf can help, but it takes a longer time to achieve your goals. Weight lifting is not recommended and should be used only after you check with your doctor, since the heart and blood pressure can respond differently to this than to walking and similar types of exercise.

Exercise is an easy and inexpensive way to greatly help your heart— you can lower your risk of heart attack and death *if* you take charge of this risk factor.

10

Between Doctor and Patient: Questions You May Have

Effective communication with your doctor could save you from heart attack. After reading this book, write down any questions you may have concerning your risk factors for heart attack or any symptoms you may have noticed, and talk with your doctor about your concerns. Once you understand how heart attack can affect your body, you can take immediate measures to prevent it from happening to you. If you have already had a heart attack, know that what you do now is important in preventing another attack later. Learn from others who have been through this, and make lifestyle changes, including a low-fat diet, exercise, stress control and more, so that your heart health is protected.

Here are answers to some of the questions we hear most frequently.

A FAMILY HISTORY OF HEART ATTACK

Q. My older brother just had a heart attack at age forty-three. He's back to work now, but I live in constant fear that I will be next. I only smoke a little, and I'm not that overweight—maybe ten pounds. What should I do? I can't sleep at night because of this fear.

A. You are smart to learn from your brother's experience, since you are definitely at higher risk for heart attack. The current guidelines by the National Cholesterol Education Program include a warning of higher risk if you have a male family member who has had a heart attack before age fifty-five or a female family member who has experienced one before age sixty-five. Since you can't change your family history, it is very important to look at your other risk factors.

For example, your smoking may be "light," but there is good evidence that one to four cigarettes per day raise the risk of coronary heart disease. Even those who don't smoke at all but are around smokers have an increased risk! (See p. 29.) Kicking the cigarette habit is one of the most treatable ways to lower your risk, even though it may be difficult at first.

You should check your other risk factors, including blood cholesterol and blood pressure, by consulting the list on p. 50. It is very important to control every risk factor you can to keep your risk at a minimum. What a great way to affect your future health! Think of the amount of time and effort you would be willing to spend if you had a heart attack. Then realize that you can spend a fraction of that time in prevention and hopefully never have the attack. The peace of mind alone is worth it.

Q. How strong is the risk factor of family history for heart attack? Both my older brothers and my father had heart attacks before age sixty. Am I next? I am forty-three years old. I watch my diet, don't smoke, have normal blood pressure, and run three miles every night.

A. Your family history is strongly positive, so you are right to be concerned now. The exact way in which our genes increase the risk of heart attack is not known, but in many cases problems are treatable. For example, if your father or your brothers had hypertension or high blood cholesterol then you should be able to overcome these problems if you yourself are at risk.

Check your own risk factors. If you take the time to work on all those under your control, you will minimize the effect of your positive family history. It might also be a good idea to consider adding vitamin E supplements.

WHAT ABOUT DIABETES?

Q. Why does having diabetes put me at risk for heart attack? I thought that had something to do with blood sugar and the pancreas. This makes no sense to me. Although I have diabetes, I don't want to worry about my heart now. Please explain.

A. It is true that in diabetes mellitus insulin produced by the pancreas is insufficient or ineffective, which results in higher blood glucose (blood sugar). This is usually treated by diet, weight control, and, at times, medications. Some diabetics require insulin to control the blood glucose (Type I), and some do not need insulin (Type II).

Diabetics have two to three times the average risk of heart attack. The longer you have diabetes, the higher the risk. While the exact causes of this increased risk are not known, it is possible that the higher levels of glucose over the years increase the damage to the inside lining of the coronary arteries. The way the body handles insulin may increase the chance of atherosclerosis. Also, HDL cholesterol is often low, and triglycerides are often high in diabetics, which both increase the risk of heart disease. When blood glucose is controlled, the cholesterol and triglycerides often improve and lower the risk of heart attack.

The best advice is to control your blood glucose as well as possible with your doctor's advice, and check your risk factors in the list on p. 51. Control other risk factors, and you can lower your risk of heart disease.

HIGHER RISK FOR WOMEN AFTER MENOPAUSE

Q. I am a 62-year-old woman with no history of heart attack in my family until now. My older sister, age seventy-eight, recently suffered a heart attack while playing golf. She was not overweight, played golf or tennis every day, and watched everything she ate. She didn't smoke, either. What went wrong? What should I do now to protect myself?

A. The risk of heart attack increases with age. The risk in women is much lower than in men until the time of menopause, but by age sixty-five women catch up. After that, the risk is roughly equal in women and men.

The risk for heart disease increases along with the blood cholesterol until at least age eighty. Although heart disease is still the most common cause of death in women and men after age sixty-five, lowering the cholesterol does seem to help.

Review your risk, especially your cholesterol level and blood pressure. Check with your doctor to see whether estrogen treatment would be right for you. Estrogen treatment after menopause lowers heart attack and other cardiovascular disease by about 40 percent. Other preventive measures such as a regular exercise program and taking vitamin E and one aspirin a day are possibilities, depending on your individual situation.

HOW TO DEAL WITH HYPERTENSION?

Q. My blood pressure is 140/80. My doctor always says that we should watch this. I'm thinking of starting a regular exercise program of walking and bike riding. Would this help bring down the top reading?

A. You should check your blood pressure as often as every few months, since it is a level at which any increase might indicate the need for treatment. The reason for controlling blood pressure is that it increases your chance of heart attack and other cardiovascular disease, which are the most common causes of serious illness and death. You can lower your own risk simply by controlling blood pressure.

What level of blood pressure is dangerous? Research shows that the risk of cardiovascular disease gradually increases with blood pressure above 120/80; if it exceeds 140/90, the risk of heart attack and other cardiovascular disease becomes high enough to need treatment.

You may want to consider treatment without medication at first. This includes a regular exercise program, so your choices of walking and bike riding are excellent. Check with your doctor to see if it's safe to begin. You may need to have an exercise test first to help make this decision.

Start slowly, walking one to two minutes per session, then gradually increase. Don't worry about how quickly you increase, it's what you do over months and years that makes the difference.

During exercise, the upper number (systolic blood pressure) may actually increase, while the lower number often decreases slightly. The benefits of a long term exercise program for you, however, may be to gradually lower the blood pressure as your physical conditioning improves.

Other ways to help reduce blood pressure without medication include decreasing your salt intake, since some people notice a drop in blood pressure when this is done. Also, if you're overweight, dieting may lower blood pressure. Check the other suggestions on pp. 83ff.

ANGIOPLASTY

Q. My father is seventy-two years old and recently had a heart attack. They did angioplasty that very night. Isn't it dangerous to perform such a drastic procedure while he is in such pain with heart attack? What is the next step for him? Will he need angioplasty each year?

A. Angioplasty (see p. 77) is a procedure in which a balloon-tipped catheter is placed directly into the blocked coronary artery. The balloon is inflated and so reduces the blockage of the artery. This is done without general anesthesia, is not painful, and may help prevent more extensive open heart surgery.

Your father received prompt treatment, and it is likely that a short length of blockage in the coronary artery was treated. In most cases, this treatment quickly improves the blood flow to the heart and may prevent further damage. About 30 percent of the time, however, the blockage returns in three to six months, usually from a blood clot in the area. Then the treatment must be repeated or the patient may need open heart coronary bypass surgery.

Angioplasty is now considered a standard treatment for this disease. Long-term results show that most patients benefit for years and many avoid open heart surgery.

As long as he does well, there is no set time at which your father would need to have angioplasty done again. Remember that he can lower his chance of future problems if he controls his risk factors for heart disease and continues his medications as advised by his doctor.

CAN BEANS HELP THE HEART?

Q. I read where eating lentils and beans can help prevent heart attack. Are there any studies that prove this? What other foods can help protect the heart?

A. Lentils and beans can be used as part of a diet to lower your intake of saturated fats, but they alone do not prevent heart attack. Meats are a good source of protein, which is a necessary part of our diet. But meats, especially red meats, contain saturated fats, which can raise the blood cholesterol. This increases the risk of heart attack.

A diet to lower saturated fats and cholesterol will probably limit your intake of meats, especially red meats. Fish, chicken, turkey or vegetables can be used to provide protein. Meats lean and carefully trimmed of fat can also be a part of the diet. Lentils, beans, and other items listed here are good sources of protein with low fat. Be sure to complement the bean dish with a grain (rice, pasta, or bread) in order to have a "complete protein." This is because legumes are high in lysine and low in tryptophan and methionine while grains are low in lysine but high in tryptophan and methionine. Taken in combination with one another, they are no different than the protein found in meat or eggs.

Legumes include: black beans, black-eyed peas, brown beans, chickpeas, Great Northern beans, kidney beans, lentils, navy beans, peas, pinto beans, red beans, and soybeans (including tofu).

Other foods may have a beneficial effect and help prevent heart disease. For example, fish such as herring and others containing *omega-3* fats help to lower the risk of heart attack by lowering triglyceride levels, and perhaps by affecting the way the body forms blood clots in the arteries. The main ingredient in fish oils, called EPA (or fish oil capsules), can be purchased separately in most drug stores or health food stores.

Monounsaturated fats such as olive oil can be used in the diet in place of saturated fats. When this is done, LDL cholesterol is lowered, which also lowers the risk of heart attack. This is a common part of the Mediterranean diet (see p. 33).

Read chapter 7 to find out more about your diet and the prevention and treatment of heart attack.

THE IMPORTANCE OF EXERCISE

Q. I am a 52-year-old attorney with most of the risk factors for heart attack—excess weight, hypertension, high cholesterol, age, being male, and lack of exercise. The good news is that I am beginning a program to reduce my risks starting today. How long will it take for my risk factors to go down?

A. You've probably accomplished the hardest part—understanding the need to lower your risk of heart attack and making the commitment to begin. Your risk will gradually diminish as your lifestyle changes.

An exercise program will help you stay fit, lose weight, and lower your blood pressure. It is a great way to begin, but you should check with your doctor; you may need an exercise test first to determine whether it is safe for your heart.

A simple walking program is discussed on p. 39. Start slowly and gradually increase, with the long-term goal being to improve your endurance and fitness. Walking briskly for about thirty minutes each day is enough to help lower your heart risk.

You'll probably first notice that your energy and the overall sense of well-being will improve. Most people find that as they exercise and lose weight, they feel better overall. Businesses find that executives and other workers are *more productive* when they exercise regularly. As a result, they find it cost-effective to make exercise equipment available in or near the workplace.

As you control each risk factor, your overall heart attack risk drops. Remember, this is a long-term plan to change your lifestyle, not simply a quick fix. Start your plan and keep to it every day, even when it may not be convenient.

THE VALUE OF VITAMIN E

Q. What are the latest studies on Vitamin E as a protector of the heart? I read that it isn't totally proven, but then all these doctors and researchers say they are taking the vitamin.

A. Vitamin E is an antioxidant—it takes up free radicals which are produced during the body's normal chemical processes. These free radicals can combine and change other compounds in the body to damage cells. For example, it is thought that cholesterol may be changed by free radicals into a form that is more damaging to arteries; this, in turn, could lead to more artery injury and atherosclerosis, including coronary artery disease. It is also possible that these free radicals are involved in other physical problems, including some forms of cancer.

Vitamin E takes up these free radicals, and although still unproven, this action might delay or stop their contribution to atherosclerosis and heart disease.

Researchers found that in a large group of men and women, vitamin E supplements of more than 100 International units (IU) per day reduced the risk of heart disease by up to one-half.

Vegetable oils contain vitamin E; however, 100 IU of vitamin E would need to be taken as a supplement, since it would be difficult to obtain that level from your diet.

WHEN IS CORONARY BYPASS SURGERY NECESSARY?

Q. How risky is coronary bypass surgery? My doctor told me that my husband, age seventy, may need to have it done. This frightens me because he seems so frail. Should I seek another opinion, and are there any other options available?

A. In coronary artery bypass graft surgery, a portion of a vein from a leg directly connects the aorta (the large artery coming from the heart) and a coronary artery. See figure 5.2.) Or, a portion of an artery from the chest (internal mammary artery) is joined to a coronary artery. The coronary artery is joined past the blockage to an area that has more normal blood flow. In other words, the blood is "rerouted" past the blockage to again supply the heart muscle.

Coronary bypass surgery is reserved for those patients who don't improve enough with medical treatment or who would not benefit from treatments such as angioplasty; or else they may show blockages that are too long or too extensive to be relieved by angioplasty. Coronary artery bypass surgery has been demonstrated to give relief in angina pectoris patients. Most studies also show improvement in chances of future heart attack and death compared to only medical treatment. Every patient is different. Your doctor, cardiologist, and cardiac surgeon can give you the best advice for your own situation.

IT'S NEVER TOO EARLY TO BEGIN
HEALTHY HEART HABITS

Q. I am a 30-year-old woman with two sons. My husband's family has a high risk for heart disease, and I want to do everything possible to protect my children. Where do I begin?

A. It is never too early to begin to prevent heart disease, and the ideal time is during childhood. Diet is one of the most important items for parents to consider, since they control what their child eats, especially in the early years. Since it is known that atherosclerosis can begin in childhood, heart risk starts in childhood, too. Since your children may be at higher risk, so it makes sense to take steps early. The dietary habits children learn at home often are those they keep as adults, even though there will probably be at least some fast foods and junk foods during the teenage and young adult years.

It may be a good idea to check your sons' blood cholesterol by the age of eight, including their LDL and HDL cholesterol and triglycerides, since each of these can be abnormal due to an inherited problem. Your doctor can guide you.

Some guidelines suggested by the World Health Organization for children two years old and above include lowering saturated fat to about 10 percent of the total calories in the child's diet if possible. Increasing the amount of monounsaturated fat (such as olive oil) is likewise recommended. If your sons have a specific cholesterol-related problem, your doctor may need to guide treatment with diet and other measures.

Hypertension happens in children, with over two million cases in the United States. Don't let this problem go unnoticed. If your sons are overweight, this should be controlled.

Many childhood habits continue into adult life. Healthy eating habits, a regular exercise program, and control of body weight should begin at home during the early years for best results.

THE TYPES OF ANGINA

Q. What is angina? How do you know if you have it? Is it dangerous?

A. Angina pectoris is discomfort in the chest caused by an insufficent blood or oxygen supply to meet the heart's demands at one time. It usually happens when the heart must do extra work, such as walking, lifting, or handling stress. Angina may be felt as squeezing, pressing, dull, aching, or sharp sensations, as discussed on p. 54. It may be accompanied by mild shortness of breath. This discomfort usually lasts for a few minutes and goes away with rest or with a nitroglycerin medication placed under the tongue or sprayed in the mouth.

The reason to notice angina pain is that it may be a sign of a serious, even life-threatening, heart problem.

There is more than one type of *angina pectoris*. *Stable angina* has not changed recently, goes away quickly, and is often predictable with certain activities (e.g., walking, working, or swimming). Most persons have a pattern of angina with which they are familiar—any change is noticeable and should be reported to your doctor.

In *unstable angina* the pattern of pain changes: it lasts longer, happens more often, or comes on more easily with less activity. Also, angina pain lasting longer than about twenty minutes is considered *unstable.*

A proper diagnosis determined mainly by talking with your doctor, who will know what characteristic signs to look for. Tests to confirm the diagnosis and to find out whether there is in fact any blockage in the coronary arteries are discussed in chapter 4.

The most dangerous type of angina is *unstable angina* or *prolonged chest pain* of more than twenty minutes' duration. The risk is higher because in these cases there may be sudden worsening and development of heart attack, with all its risks, including sudden death. If angina becomes unstable or prolonged chest discomfort occurs, you should contact your doctor immediately. There are many other causes of chest discomfort that may mimic angina, but it is not safe to guess the answer without medical evaluation!

HANDLING STRESS

Q. How does stress relate to the heart? I am a 45-year-old air traffic controller—the job with the highest reported stress. Now I'm worried not only about my job each day, but how my job is affecting my heart. Can you give me some tips to reduce my worries and stress?

A. Yes, stress can affect the heart, causing hypertension, overeating, and excess weight. Stress can also cause fatigue, which limits activity and exercise; it may also produce changes in the body as discussed in chapter 8, which increase the risk of heart disease.

Those with other high-stress jobs, such as bus drivers in large cities, have been found to have higher stress levels, greater risk of heart disease, and higher overall death rates. Job strain (its demands and the ability to control those demands) can be high in any job, including yours. Studies also show that workers who feel they are under higher stress in their jobs have a higher risk of heart disease.

What can you do? Read chapter 8 dealing with stress and the heart, and try to identify which specific areas of your work and other aspects of your life are the main sources of stress. Then use the techniques suggested to control the stress in your life. If you don't feel any improvement, it would be a good idea to talk to a specialist in dealing in effective stress management, such as a clinical psychologist or psychiatrist. We can't eliminate all the stress we have, but we can definitely control how we respond to it!

Additional Reading

Suggestions for additional reading are listed. A complete list of references is available from the authors through the publisher.

National High Blood Pressure Program. *The Fifth Report of the Joint National Committee on Detection, Evaluation and Treatment of High Blood Pressure.* Washington, D.C.: National Institutes of Health; National Institutes of Heart, Lung, and Blood. January 1993.

The Heart, Arteries and Veins. Ed. J. Willis Hurst, M.D. New York: McGraw-Hill, 1990.

National Heart, Lung and Blood Institute Data Fact Sheet. Morbidity from Coronary Heart Disease in the United States. May 1992.

National High Blood Pressure Education Program Working Group on Primary Prevention of Hypertension. Washington, D.C.: National Institutes of Health; National Institutes of Heart, Lung, and Blood. May 1993.

Report of the Expert Panel on Population Strategies for Blood Cholesterol Reduction. Executive Summary. Washington, D.C.: U.S. Department of Health and Human Services; Public Health Service; National Institutes of Health; National Institutes of Heart, Lung, and Blood; National Cholesterol Education Program. March 1993.

Second Report of the Expert Panel on Detection, Evaluation and Treatment of High Blood Cholesterol in Adults. Washington, D.C.: National Institutes of Health; National Institutes of Heart, Lung, and Blood. September 1993.